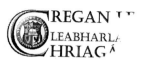

Critical Psychiatry

Critical Psychiatry

The Limits of Madness

Edited by

D. B. Double

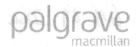

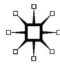

First published 2006 by
PALGRAVE MACMILLAN
Houndmills, Basingstoke, Hampshire RG21 6XS and
175 Fifth Avenue, New York, N. Y. 10010
Companies and representatives throughout the world

PALGRAVE MACMILLAN is the global academic imprint of the Palgrave Macmillan division of St. Martin's Press, LLC and of Palgrave Macmillan Ltd. Macmillan® is a registered trademark in the United States, United Kingdom and other countries. Palgrave is a registered trademark in the European Union and other countries.

ISBN-13: 978–0–230–00128–2 hardback
ISBN-10: 0–230–00128–9 hardback

This book is printed on paper suitable for recycling and made from fully managed and sustained forest sources.

A catalogue record for this book is available from the British Library.

Library of Congress Cataloging-in-Publication Data
Critical psychiatry: the limits of madness / edited by D. B. Double.
    p. cm.
  Includes bibliographical references and index.
  ISBN 0–230–00128–9 (cloth)
    1. Psychiatry—Philosophy. 2. Mental health policy. 3. Crisis intervention (Mental health services) 4. Psychiatry—Social aspects.
  I. Double, D.B., 1952–

RC437.5.C75 2006
616.89—dc22

2006042587

10   9   8   7   6   5   4   3   2
15   14   13   12   11   10   09

Printed and bound in Great Britain b
Antony Rowe Ltd, Chippenham and

Man is most often led from the free use of reason to madness by over-stepping the limits of his good qualities and of his generous and magnanimous inclinations.

Phillippe Pinel, 'Memoir on madness', 11 December, 1794

Truth has its limits, absurdity has none.

Ernst von Feuchtersleben, *The principles of medical psychology*, 1845

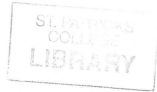

Contents

List of Tables and Figures   ix

Notes on Contributors   xi

Introduction

1   Critical Psychiatry: Challenging the Biomedical   3
    Dominance of Psychiatry
    D.B. Double

Part I: Anti-psychiatry and Critical Psychiatry in Retrospect

2   Historical Perspectives on Anti-psychiatry   19
    D.B. Double

3   From Anti-psychiatry to Critical Psychiatry   41
    John M. Heaton

4   Transcultural Mental Health Care: The Challenge   61
    to Positivist Psychiatry
    David Ingleby

Part II: The Prospect of Critical Psychiatry

5   The Limits of Biomedical Models of Distress   81
    Lucy Johnstone

6   Understanding Psychiatry's Resistance to Change   99
    Terry Lynch

7   The Politics of Psychiatric Drug Treatment   115
    Joanna Moncrieff

8   British Mental Health Social Work and the Psychosocial   133
    Approach in Context
    Shulamit Ramon

9 Democracy, Citizenship and the Radical Possibilities   149
   of Postpsychiatry
   Pat Bracken & Philip Thomas

10 The Biopsychological Approach in Psychiatry: 165
    The Meyerian Legacy
    D.B. Double

11 Critical Child Psychiatry   189
    Sami Timimi

Conclusion

12 Critical Psychiatry and Conflict: Renewing   209
    Mental Health Practice
    D.B. Double

References   227

Index   249

List of Tables

Table 7.1   Results of the Finnish Minimal Use Study   131

List of Figures

Figure 2.1   Subdivisions of Anti-psychiatry   31
Figure 9.1   The Emergence of Psychiatry from the Age of Reason   152
Figure 10.1   Meyer's Understanding of Science   175

Notes on Contributors

Pat Bracken is clinical director of the West Cork Mental Health Services, Ireland. He is co-editor of *Rethinking the trauma of war* (London: Free Association, 1998), author of *Trauma: Culture, meaning and philosophy* (London: Whurr Publishers, 2002) and co-author of *Postpsychiatry: Mental health in a postmodern world* (Oxford: OUP, 2005).

D.B. Double is consultant psychiatrist and honorary senior lecturer, Norfolk and Waveney Mental Health Partnership NHS Trust and University of East Anglia. He is website editor of the Critical Psychiatry Network (www.criticalpsychiatry.co.uk).

John M. Heaton is a psychotherapist and one-time colleague of R.D. Laing. He is the author of *Wittgenstein and psychoanalysis* (Duxford: Icon Books, 2000)

David Ingleby is professor of intercultural psychology, Utrecht University, the Netherlands. He is the editor of *Critical psychiatry: The politics of mental health* (Harmondsworth: Penguin, 1981) and *Forced migration and mental health: Rethinking the care of refugees and displaced persons* (Springer-Verlag, 2004).

Lucy Johnstone is clinical lecturer on the doctoral programme in clinical psychology at the University of the West of England. She is the author of *Users and abusers of psychiatry: A critical look at traditional psychiatric practice* (2nd edition) (London: Routledge, 2000).

Terry Lynch is a medical practitioner and psychotherapist in Limerick and author of *Beyond Prozac: Healing mental suffering without drugs* (Ross-on-Wye: PCCS Books, 2004).

Joanna Moncrieff is senior lecturer in social and community psychiatry, University College London, Department of Psychiatry & Behavioural Sciences.

Shulamit Ramon is professor of interprofessional health and social studies, Anglia Polytechnic University, UK. Her most recent edited books are *Users researching health and social care: An empowering agenda.*

(Birmingham: Venture Press, 2003) and *Mental health at the crossroads. The promise of the psychosocial approach* (Aldershot: Ashgate, 2005).

Philip Thomas is senior research fellow at the Centre for Citizenship & Community Mental Health, University of Bradford. He is author of *The dialectics of schizophrenia* (London: Free Association, 1997) and co-author of *Voices of reason, voices of insanity: Studies of verbal hallucinations* (London: Brunner-Routledge, 2000) and *Postpsychiatry: Mental health in a postmodern world* (Oxford: OUP, 2005).

Sami Timimi is consultant child and adolescent psychiatrist, Lincolnshire Partnership NHS Trust. He is the author of *Pathological child psychiatry and the medicalization of childhood* (Hove: Brunner-Routledge, 2002) and *Naughty boys: Anti-social behaviour, ADHD and the role of culture* (Basingstoke: Palgrave Macmillan, 2005).

Introduction

1

Critical Psychiatry: Challenging the Biomedical Dominance of Psychiatry

D.B. Double

The first modern use of the term 'critical psychiatry' was probably in *Critical psychiatry: The politics of mental health*, an edited book by David Ingleby (1980a). This book has recently been reissued by Free Association Books (2004). The new publisher's blurb suggests that far from being merely a historical document, the book is powerfully relevant to mental health services today. The book makes a strong plea for critical thinking about the conceptual foundations of psychiatry, about its social role, and about the issues of power surrounding mental illness.

The first chapter of *Critical psychiatry*, entitled 'Understanding mental illness', was written by Ingleby (1980b) himself and forms about a third of the book. The chapter critiques the dominant, mainstream biological approach in psychiatry for its overly positivist stance, and instead promotes an alternative interpretative paradigm. In a review of the book in *New Society*, Peter Sedgwick (1981) commented that 'the interpretative, anti-scientistic arguments produced by David Ingleby ... deserve an airing'. This sentiment very much agrees with this present book, and these issues will be discussed further in its various chapters.

Sedgwick also noted that Ingleby had failed to obtain a tenured lectureship at Cambridge University for which Sedgwick had provided a testimonial. Sedgwick's reference was favourable and was partly based on his evaluation of the introductory editorial article and opening chapter for *Critical psychiatry*, which had been part of the evidence presented to the referees. However, rumours claimed that Ingleby had been turned down because of adverse (indeed hostile) reports from his referees. It is commonly supposed that the hostile report was from Martin Roth, professor of psychiatry in Cambridge at the time and a figure of national eminence, having been the first president of the Royal College of

Psychiatrists (see chapter 4 for David Ingleby's own account of this incident).

On hearing of Ingleby's difficulties in securing tenure every single one of his colleagues in the Social and Political Sciences Committee signed a letter regretting the appointments committee's decision. In 1980, Ingleby had his second application for upgrading refused by the University. The treatment of David Ingleby stimulated a large and vocal undergraduate protest. In 1982, he moved to Holland to take up a chair in Developmental Psychology at Utrecht University.

Ingleby found a sympathetic social climate in the Netherlands. By the end of the seventies, Holland had become a byword for liberalism and progressive social policies (Ingleby, 1998). However, over recent years, as Ingleby himself notes, 'there has been a noticeable shift ... away from socially critical perspectives, which are increasingly regarded as an embarrassing hangover from the seventies'. The message of critical psychiatry has become lost in the highly bureaucratic and rationalised state of modern mental health services.

This state of affairs seems timely for a re-statement of critical psychiatry, and this book is intended to provide just such an account. Far from believing that critical psychiatry is merely tied to the liberal social perspective of the 1960s, this book recognises the enduring nature of the debate about mental disorder. Ever since society, in the form of the state, first accepted responsibility for caring for the mentally ill by building asylums, our understanding of mental illness has remained caught in metaphysical questions about the nature of reality. The issues of critical psychiatry are therefore not new. Essentially the problem is the connection between mind and matter and the way it impinges on the relationship between facts and values. This book's aim is to approach this fundamental issue afresh.

The relationship between critical psychiatry and anti-psychiatry

The title of this book *Critical psychiatry: The limits of madness* deliberately echoes the original book by Ingleby. It has very similar aims. It resolutely encourages critical thinking about psychiatry and is based on critical theory about the nature of psychiatry.

Yet my book is written at a different time. Ingleby's book appeared at the end of a turbulent period of cultural criticism of psychiatry, commonly recognised as 'anti-psychiatry' (see chapter 2). This critique, perhaps best identified with the names of R.D. Laing and Thomas Szasz, is generally viewed as a passing phase in the history of psychiatry (Tantam, 1991). It is said to be no longer of any influence. The modern version of critical psychiatry described in my book is, therefore, 'post-anti-psychiatry', in the sense that it is being presented again in the relative calm of a period when there has been time to reflect on the impact of anti-psychiatry.

It is important to place anti-psychiatry in its broader cultural context and see it in terms of its continuities as well as discontinuities (Gijswijt-Hofstra & Porter, 1998). It is hardly surprising that Martin Roth was opposed to David Ingleby. For example, he wrote, with Jerome Kroll, the book *The reality of mental illness* (Roth & Kroll, 1986) which was written to counter anti-psychiatry. As was generally the case, critiques of psychiatry, including Ingleby's, were lumped together as anti-psychiatry and dismissed for this reason. Because of this rejection, Roth may not have fully appreciated, unlike Sedgwick in his book review, that Ingleby's position is 'free from the Laingian and Szaszian excesses which have given anti-psychiatry such a rotten reputation'.

Martin Roth's banishment of Ingleby represents the marginalisation of critical psychiatry. In the next chapter of this book, I provide a history of anti-psychiatry and give more detail about its nature and viewpoints. This chapter, in providing a historical account, aims to provide a basis for elucidating the differences between critical psychiatry and anti-psychiatry. These terms are not always used very precisely. In fact, 'anti-psychiatry' is a general label that has tended to be used by the psychiatric mainstream to identify its opposition. Both Laing and Szasz rejected the designation of themselves.

What I am suggesting is that although critical psychiatry has its roots in anti-psychiatry, it does represent an advance over the polarisation in the debate about psychiatry engendered by anti-psychiatry. In fact, the term anti-psychiatry, in combining such conflicting viewpoints as those of Laing and Szasz, does not do justice to the differing foundations of the critique. Also, anti-psychiatry, at least in its Laingian version, may have ultimately been more interested in personal liberation and spiritual growth. This may have contributed to it becoming a 'dead-end' in the history of psychiatry. Laing's quest for personal authenticity meant he was not interested or able to carry through his ideas to change psychiatry professionally. He became trapped in his training in psychotherapy, part of it undertaken at the Tavistock clinic, and could not return to practice in mainstream general psychiatry. As he said himself, 'What I didn't bank on, what I hadn't realised was that the Tavistock was an exclusively *out-patient* organisation' [his emphasis] (Mullan, 1995: 147). He wanted to pursue his work with more profoundly disturbed people in hospital in an inpatient setting. Once he had become infamous, it was difficult for him to return to the mainstream.

I give more detail about the history of anti-psychiatry in chapter 2. It is important to recognise that what has been labelled as anti-psychiatry covers a broad church of varying opinions. There is a sense in which it is difficult to distil its essence, apart from its opposition to an overly biomedical perspective. The message of critical psychiatry is that it is possible to practice psychiatry without the justification of postulating brain pathology as the basis for mental illness. Anti-psychiatry perhaps found it more difficult to justify the practice of psychiatry in itself, or at least that was the perceived threat from the orthodox perspective.

The rest of the book takes up these aspects of critical psychiatry and anti-psychiatry. At this point, I just want to make clear what I mean when I say that anti-psychiatry became more interested in personal growth and authenticity than changing psychiatry. As an example, I would mention Jan Foudraine, who was very much identified with anti-psychiatry. In his notoriety, he could be seen as the Dutch equivalent of the British psychiatrist and 'anti-psychiatrist', R.D. Laing. His bestselling book *Not made of wood* (Foudraine, 1974), as it was entitled in English translation, still figures on many people's list of 'books that have influenced my life'. The book describes Foudraine's disappointment as an assistant-psychiatrist with the lack of 'human dignity' in traditional psychiatric practice. He was also frustrated with the approach of Chestnut Lodge in Rockville, Maryland, USA, a psychiatric hospital which became renowned for its intensive psychoanalytic treatment of psychosis, associated with distinguished staff, such as Frieda Fromm-Reichman. Foudraine worked there for a few years, transforming his ward into a 'school for life'.

Foudraine admitted he was confused by the reaction to his best-selling book. He became the 'personal ambassador' in Holland of Bhagwan Shree Rajneesh. Osho, as he later came to be called, was an Indian spiritual leader who preached an eclectic doctrine of Eastern mysticism, individual devotion and sexual freedom while amassing vast personal wealth.

At a talk that Foudraine gave at a Critical Psychiatry Network conference in Sheffield in 2001, he advised giving up the struggle against the biomedical dominance of psychiatry. Instead he suggested that 'the belief in a "me" as a separate entity … is the real problem underlying and structuring all of our problems' (Foudraine, 2001). In his own words,

Eastern mystics have told us that the world indeed is 'maya', illusory. … Instead of fighting the medical model I became much more interested in 'maya' or the prison of conceptualising, and the core of 'maya' being the belief in a separate 'me'.

This philosophical position should be respected and valued as a legitimate stance on the issues posed by critical psychiatry. It should not necessarily be dismissed as mere romanticism. After all, both Eastern philosophy and postmodernism could be said to coincide in their recognition of the lack of fixity of the individual's sense of a centred self. Deconstruction may be said to have its origins in Nietsche's contention that there are no facts, only interpretations – or in Foudraine's words, 'What we are doing is continuously interpreting what the senses are offering us'. There are genuine problems about the nature of knowledge that do need to be considered seriously, even if we do not necessarily agree with Foudraine's solution.

The next chapter (chapter 3) is written by John Heaton, who was also intimately involved in the origins of 'anti-psychiatry', in that he was an early colleague of R.D. Laing. Heaton is still a leading figure in the Philadelphia Association (www.philadelphia-association.co.uk) which was originally set up by Laing and others as a charitable organisation to 'change the way the "facts" of "mental health" and "mental illness" are seen' (Cooper, 1994). The organisation eventually disowned Laing as its Chairman, and still continues to provide several therapeutic community households and psychotherapy training courses in London.

In his chapter, Heaton emphasises the liberatory nature of anti-psychiatry and discusses the nature of human freedom. He suggests that critical psychiatry is a practice that states frankly what one thinks about the nature of persons and psychiatry. He utilises the notion of *parrhesia* from Foucault's later books to understand the relation of oneself to the truth. In this respect, he criticises both psychoanalysis and cognitive therapy. Again, using the later Foucauldian term *genealogy*, first used by Nietsche, he describes the illusory nature of the objectivity created by the power and knowledge of psychiatry and psychoanalysis.

Heaton's contribution to this book is very welcome and reminds us of the philosophical contribution of Laing as a major critic of orthodox, medically based psychiatry (Collier, 1977). The Philadelphia Association does not subscribe to a particular theoretical model or school, but utilises philosophy, particularly phenomenology, existentialism, the sceptical philosophies and psychoanalytic thought, to think about mental life and question the cultural norms and assumptions that may be implicit in a person's suffering or accepted ways of understanding it. As noted by Heaton, an important practice of Laing's was to have a copy of one or other of a well-known critical theoretical text in the therapeutic community households – Merleau-Ponty and some Buddhist texts were the most popular. The point of this was not to turn people into amateur philosophers but to remind them that 'there is a long and distinguished tradition of thought about the human condition which is far greater than the narrow positivism of psychoanalysis and modern psychiatry'. The early and 'middle' work of Foucault has been widely discussed in relation to mental health. Heaton takes this analysis forward in his chapter by also making connections with Foucault's later work, which has a more positive understanding of human freedom.

In the next chapter (chapter 4), David Ingleby describes how he later became involved in the field of transcultural mental health after the publication of *Critical psychiatry* (Ingleby, 1981). He relates issues of ethnicity, cultural diversity and globalisation to critical psychiatry, even though questions of race and culture did not figure prominently in the original debates of the 1960s and 70s. He also reinforces the distinction he first made in his chapter in *Critical psychiatry* between positivist and interpretative approaches to mental health, which he suggests are 'two components of the mentality that characterises European thinking since the Enlightenment'. The interculturalisation of mental health overlaps with many of the issues of critical psychiatry, such as the importance of social context in the understanding of people's mental problems and criticism of the unwarranted medicalisation of these problems.

Interestingly, as previously mentioned, Ingleby notes the backlash against the social cultural critiques of the 1960s and 70s. He relates part of the reason for this change to a shift from a neo-Marxist perspective to poststructuralism. The concept of power, for example as used by Foucault, placed an emphasis on the discourse of psychiatry. For whatever reasons, the demise of critical approaches led to 'an increasingly monolithic grip of positivistic orthodoxy' on mental health theory and practice.

The restatement of critical psychiatry

The first three chapters in this book, after the introduction, all have an aspect of looking back at the history of anti-psychiatry. John Heaton and David Ingleby were both intimately involved in the earlier debates. The subsequent chapters are written by people who can be seen as part of the fresh wave of critical psychiatry. Many are prominent figures in what can be seen as a new movement, re-establishing a critical base for psychiatric practice.

The first of these authors is Lucy Johnstone (chapter 5), known for her inspiring book *Users and abusers of psychiatry* (Johnstone, 2000). After the second edition of this book, Johnstone returned from an academic post to practice as a clinical psychologist. She had felt she had to leave clinical work because she was hounded for her dissenting views. Her return to clinical work shows that her stance does not come from mere 'ivory tower' theorising. Her book describes how mainstream psychiatry, contrary to its apparent intentions, fails to address emotional problems. From her perspective, in fact it compounds the difficulties by rescuing people with a medical label, encouraging them to rely on an external solution that is rarely forthcoming. In her book she undermines the evidence for the medical model in a passionate and forceful way.

Johnstone's chapter in this book elaborates her critique of the biomedical paradigm. She points out that psychiatric diagnosis involves social judgements lacking medical objectivity. She critiques the notions commonly adopted by psychiatrists in clinical practice of biochemical imbalance and genetic causation in mental illness. She raises the intriguing question of how and why biomedical theories survive despite the lack of evidence. These arguments are basic to the position of critical psychiatry.

The next chapter (chapter 6) by Terry Lynch specifically addresses the question of why psychiatry is so resistant to change. As he notes, doctors commonly believe that people who are mentally unwell have a chemical imbalance in the brain, without the existence of any test that could possibly verify this hypothesis. Professional insecurity encourages them to take this step of faith. To admit it is false would mean losing face to such a degree that they would feel their respectability and status are seriously undermined. Mental illness is clearly not the same sort of disorder as diabetes, as some doctors claim, if only because psychological treatments, including placebo effects, are important. Prescribing medication is based on a biased overinterpretation of the evidence. Patients do find psychosocial interventions helpful. These points reinforce the case for critical psychiatry.

Lynch is known for his book *Beyond Prozac: Healing mental suffering without drugs* (Lynch, 2001), which was a bestseller in Ireland. He trained and practised as a GP before becoming a psychotherapist. It is GPs who initiate most prescribing in mental health and other disorders. Their attitude to critical psychiatry is important.

The chapter that follows is by Joanna Moncrieff (chapter 7). It critiques the evidence-base for the use of psychotropic drugs. Critical psychiatry may be different from anti-psychiatry in being prepared to debate the evidence with mainstream psychiatry. It is all very well to dismiss physical treatments, as did much of anti-psychiatry, but such treatments are justified by the results of clinical trials. Critical psychiatry engages with the data and highlights the extent to which its interpretation is generally biased in favour of treatment. There may still be a sense in which it is impossible to prove beyond any reasonable doubt that medication and other treatments are effective, and this, for example, was Sigmund Freud's position, at least as regards psychoanalysis. Nonetheless it is important that the data is evaluated in an unbiased way. In fact, clinical trials are often claimed to provide a scientific basis for claims for efficacy, but science demands a sceptical and impartial assessment, and this element is often lacking.

Moncrieff summarises the basic critique of the data on antipsychotic medication, lithium and other drugs for bipolar disorder (manic-depressive illness), and antidepressants. She then goes on to examine how the vested interests of three powerful social groups: the pharmaceutical industry, the psychiatric profession and the state, have worked to promote the use of drugs for psychological disorders. As mentioned previously, perhaps of particular interest is the role of psychiatrists themselves in defending the biomedical system to buttress their status. Physical treatments create a sense of optimism amongst professionals, but the problem is that this emphasis avoids the hard work necessary to help people make real changes to their lives. It is difficult to deny the extent to which psychiatry is a social practice, and governments have been enticed by the potential social control available to psychiatry. This is evident in the reports from the 1960s and 70s that the authorities in the Soviet Union were incarcerating substantial numbers of dissidents in mental asylums.

Perhaps not of the same degree, but there is a similar risk in the current reforms of the Mental Health Act 1983. For example, preventive detention of people with so-called Dangerously Severe Personality Disorder (DSPD) could be seen as the government's attempt to introduce such provision by the backdoor in the mental health system rather than seeking to justify it in the criminal system. The motivation for reform of the Act was to ensure that 'patients get supervised care if they do not take their medication or if their condition deteriorates' (Department of Health, 1998a). This government statement could be seen as reflecting a naïve assessment of the value of psychotropic medication. The thought seems to be that all that is needed to avoid disaster is that patients should continue to take their medication. Yet a psychiatric profession that should know better has tended to encourage such oversimplification. Joanna Moncrieff is very clear about the political nature of psychiatric drug treatment. More specifically, she raises the question that should commonly be asked, and rarely is, as to whether people may gain more benefit in the long-term from working through their personal and social problems without psychotropic medication. Far too much of the emphasis in assessment in clinical trials is on short-term outcome.

Chapter 8 is written by Shulamit Ramon. Although she takes an interdisciplinary approach in her research in health and social care, it is useful to have the specific viewpoint from social work that she takes. As she says, 'historically the social work perspective offered a contextualised and holistic approach to mental ill health'. Many social workers in the past would have gone along with the anti-psychiatry critique, whereas these days they are less prepared to challenge the medical dominance of psychiatry. This may well be because of the statutory responsibility that the role of Approved Social Worker imposes under the Mental Health Act 1983. Ramon argues that social workers should not necessarily feel threatened by the reform proposed amongst others in the current review of the Act that other professionals also should be able to take on the responsibility of making an application under the Act. If social work was less tied to its statutory responsibilities, the profession may again be free to take up its social model of mental illness.

The social perspective is more than a concern with the practical issues that may impact on a person's life, such as welfare benefits and housing. The Social Perspectives Network (SPN) (www.spn.org.uk) was formed in 2002 to bring together service users, carers, practitioners, educators, policy makers and researchers to promote the value of social models in today's mental health services. The key characteristics of the social model have been discussed by Duggan (2002a). These principles have been developed to understand and work with people with mental distress (Tew, 2005). Reconstruction of the psychosocial approach promises a contextualised and holistic approach to mental health problems (Ramon & Williams, 2005). Critical psychiatry is part of this social perspective.

Over recent years, Pat Bracken and Phil Thomas (2001, 2005) have promoted a new approach to mental health, which they call 'postpsychiatry'. We are fortunate that they have provided a synopsis of this viewpoint in their chapter (chapter 9). Postpsychiatry sees the modernist agenda of psychiatry as no longer tenable because of various postmodern challenges to its basis. These include questioning simple notions of progress and scientific expertise. The rise of the user movement, with its challenge to the biomedical model of mental illness, is seen as being of particular importance. Recent government policy emphases on social exclusion and partnership in health are viewed as an opportunity for a new deal between professionals and service users. Postpsychiatry is, therefore, context-centred and takes its philosophical foundations from 'hermeneutical' philosophers such as Wittgenstein and Heidegger and the Russian psychologist Vygotsky. Such approaches give priority to meaning and interpretation rather than causal explanation.

One way of understanding postpsychiatry is that postmodernism is being promoted as the basis for critical psychiatry. In fact, I think there is a debate about how much critical psychiatry needs to be tied to postmodernism. My own view is that the link with postmodernism is unnecessary and perhaps unfortunate, because critiques of postmodernism tend to conclude, for example, that it degenerates into the irrational. Not that I do not think it is important, as mooted by David Ingleby, to disentangle the impact of poststructuralism on critical psychiatry.

My own stance is that there has always been a strand of biopsychological thinking in modern psychiatry at least since the 19th century. Biomedical and biopsychological paradigms have their origins at about the same time (c. 1845) and have been in competition since then, with the biomedical in the ascendancy, although there have been times when mainstream views have been more pluralistic. I discuss these issues in chapter 10 on the biopsychological approach in psychiatry, which is particularly associated with the psychobiology of Adolf Meyer, perhaps the most eminent American psychiatrist of the first half of the 20th century. The biopsychological perspective has a long history if it is the foundation of critical psychiatry. It needs to be clearly restated in a post-anti-psychiatric age. Meyer may not have succeeded in establishing his system for various reasons, such as his tendency to express himself poorly and by compromising with other views. Critical psychiatry does need to have a cutting edge to avoid marginalisation.

Chapter 11 is written by Sami Timmi on critical child psychiatry. There are specific issues for critical psychiatry in this field. Traditionally children were regarded as not being subject to many of the mental illnesses of adults. However, child and family studies have not been immune from the developments in biomedical psychiatry over recent years. In particular, where once it was the case that medication had a very limited role in child psychiatry, it now has an increasing role, even if still restricted in the context of family and behavioural therapies. Neurological and biochemical explanations of childhood problems are now widely accepted and popularised. For example, Ritalin (methylphenidate) has been increasingly prescribed for attention-deficit/hyperactivity disorder (ADHD). Studies that purport to show that people suffering from depression have imbalances of chemicals, such as serotonin, in their brains are said to apply as much to children as adults. For instance, the American Psychiatric Association's (1998) public information leaflet on childhood depression encourages the speculation that 'an imbalance in serotonin may cause the sleep problems, irritability and anxiety characteristic of depression, while an imbalance of norepinephrine, which regulates alertness and arousal, may contribute to the fatigue and depressed mood of the illness'. Even claims for biochemical effects underlying depression in adults rarely go this far.

Timimi reinforces the hypothetical nature of these developments. It is a pity that the discipline of child psychiatry has now become so invaded by the biomedical model. Historically, the speciality of child psychiatry served as a haven and opportunity for those who wanted to escape the reductionism of their colleagues in adult psychiatry. This more holistic approach to personal and social problems is being undermined, and Timimi is determined to try to reverse this trend.

Timimi proposes that a perceived crisis of a social and moral nature in Western countries, in relation to the cultural task of child rearing, is an important factor behind the trend of medicalising social problems. Some may think that this is too grand a theory to explain the development. Nonetheless, Timimi is also concerned with the more nitty-gritty, political nature of market exploitation of children's emotional problems by drug companies, as was Joanna Moncrieff for adults in her chapter. Timimi sees this area as 'doctors carving out new and increasing roles for themselves together with aggressive marketing by the drug industry, a very powerful and difficult to resist combination'. He also provides a summary critique of the evidence against the use of Ritalin in ADHD and antidepressants for so-called 'childhood depression'.

My final chapter (chapter 12) concludes this book. It discusses the degree to which critical psychiatry is in conflict with mainstream psychiatry. Critical psychiatry does not want to be marginalised, as was anti-psychiatry. By way of summary, I attempt to define critical psychiatry, describe the key issues and clarify how critical psychiatry differs from mainstream psychiatry. These topics have been taken up in more detail in the rest of the chapters of the book.

I think it would be a mistake to regard this book as merely a restatement of the old arguments of anti-psychiatry. Of course this will be said, possibly with the unconscious motivation of wanting to deflect its challenge to mainstream psychiatry. This book is a genuine attempt to propose a new synthesis that is within the remit of psychiatry. Critical psychiatry does not want to exclude or be excluded from psychiatric practice. On the other hand, it would also be misleading to conclude that critical psychiatry is afraid of confrontation with biological psychiatry. Its aim is to gain acceptance of a pluralism within psychiatry. Besides this objective, it does look for recognition of the validity of its own position.

Is critical psychiatry a threat?

It has been suggested that the differences from mainstream psychiatry do not amount to very much and that critical psychiatry is merely an attempt to practice psychiatry more humanely. Actually I do not think this element should be belittled. However, I do agree that too much can be made of the differences. Of course I recognise the good intentions of people working in the mental health field who are not critical psychiatrists. The personal nature of psychiatry, and medicine in general, understandably creates defensive practice. I do not want to cast unnecessary blame on those that are trying to do the best for their patients. On the other hand, I do believe that the conceptual model of mental illness adopted does affect practice. Critical psychiatry explicitly confronts the tendency to objectify people and there are real advantages in this stance.

Moreover, mainstream psychiatry can find critical psychiatry threatening. I have directly experienced this through being suspended by my NHS Trust for 6 months (Double, 2004a). I had always prided myself on being able to practise psychiatry differently without causing confrontation. It was a shock to me for my employers to turn against me and to accuse me of unsafe practice. In my naïvety I never thought this could happen.

At the time I was working in a hard-pressed service, and in these circumstances the standards of practice can 'fray at the edges'. However, despite this, I do not think my standards were at any time any less than is the case in many such hard-pressed, or even less hard-pressed, services in other areas.

Moreover it is clear that there was an ideological element to the suspension. I was told I would be sent for retraining in organic psychiatry, presumably because I was thought to be deficient in this area, which is nonsense. The assessors from the Royal College of Psychiatrists, who produced a report on my practice, gave feedback that if I did not accept that I needed a period of supervision then my philosophy about psychiatry would need to be examined and my scepticism about the use of psychotropic medication challenged. Although none of these things happened, it is difficult to think they were not motivating factors in my suspension. When the College report was finally produced, I was told I needed to change but was not told how I needed to change!

Is my scepticism about psychotropic medication beyond the pale? Belief in such treatment seems to be an edifice that does not like to be attacked. But if there is such a flimsy foundation for biomedical psychiatry, why should we have faith in it? As mentioned above, placebo effects with medication can be powerful. Maybe this non-specific effect is all that is being achieved with medication. There may be no specific effect due to an active ingredient. If so, then there should be no pretence that such medication is better than placebo. We should not deceive our patients, although some doctors do not necessarily consider this intention unethical (Oh, 1994). And if patients know that psychotropic medication is merely placebo, would they take it? Understandably many people who present to mental health services are desperate and will do whatever it takes to find relief. It may well suit them to believe that medication will be helpful. But if the doctor knows that it is no better than placebo, he/she is exploiting the patient in his/her crisis. Critical psychiatry is trying to rid mental health practice of such exploitation.

The rest of the book takes up these themes. The aim is that by the end of the book you will be able to decide for yourself whether critical psychiatry is really such a threat. In my view, the book will have succeeded if it makes plain the self-deception, albeit unconscious, of much of biomedical psychiatry, and encourages instead a more open practice. However difficult the task of helping people with mental health problems may be, this book encourages the engagement of mental health professionals with these problems. The hope is that the outcome for users of services will be improved.

Part I

Anti-psychiatry and Critical Psychiatry in Retrospect

2
Historical Perspectives on Anti-psychiatry

D.B. Double

The origin of anti-psychiatry

The origin of the modern use of the term anti-psychiatry was in a book by David Cooper (1967) entitled *Psychiatry and anti-psychiatry*. In the preface, he talked about anti-psychiatry being at a germinal stage. He suggested that what he called the 'in-stitutionalising processes' and 'day-to-day indoctrination' of work in the psychiatric field were starting to produce answers antithetical to conventional solutions.

In particular, he saw schizophrenia as a label applied to people whose acts, statements and experience have been socially invalidated, so that as patients they conform to a passive, inert identity. Psychiatry was therefore seen as reinforcing the alienated needs of society. Cooper was convinced that 'the process whereby someone becomes a designated schizophrenic involves a subtle, psychological, mythical, mystical, spiritual violence'. This violence commences in the family and is perpetuated in the psychiatric hospital. He even went as far as to suggest that 'it is often when people start to become *sane* that they enter the mental hospital' [his emphasis].

Cooper, therefore, tentatively transformed psychiatry into anti-psychiatry by inverting notions of sanity and insanity. He wanted to create a community in which patients would have the chance to discover and explore authentic relatedness to others. To do this required positive non-action, 'an effort to cease interference, to "lay off" other people and give them and oneself a chance'. Being allowed to 'go to pieces' was necessary before one could be helped to come together again. He contrasted his approach with the psychiatric therapeutic community movement pioneered by Maxwell Jones (1952).

He set up Villa 21 in Shenley Hospital between January 1962 and April 1966. An experimental phase of staff withdrawal led to rubbish accumulating in the corridors and dining room tables being covered with the previous days' unwashed plates. Some staff controls were re-introduced with the threat of discharge if patients did not conform to the rules. These apparent limits to institutional change led to the conclusion that a successful unit could only be developed in the community rather than the hospital. Cooper was involved as part of the Philadelphia Association in setting up Kingsley Hall, a 'counterculture' centre in the east end of London (see below under R.D. Laing).

Cooper's theoretical perspective was built on earlier family studies of schizophrenia that attempted to characterise the predominant traits of parents of schizophrenic people. In the initial studies, mothers were seen as characteristically emotionally manipulative, dominating, over-protective and yet at the same time rejecting; fathers were characteristically weak, passive, preoccupied, ill, or, in some other sense 'absent' as an effective parent. In particular, Cooper utilised the theory of Bateson et al (1956) about the role of the double-bind manoeuvre. In this situation, parents convey two or more conflicting and incompatible messages at the same time. As the child is involved in an intense relationship, s/he feels that the communication must be understood but is unable to comment on the inconsistency because it meets with disapproval from the parents. Schizophrenia is, therefore, not to be understood as a disease entity but as a set of person-interactional patterns that require demystification of the confusion of the double-bind.

Families at Villa 21 were studied by participant observation and tape-recording of group situations with families and of the patient in ward groups. Laing & Esterson (1964) used similar techniques. As far as Cooper was concerned, the research succeeded in making the apparently absurd symptoms of schizophrenia intelligible. The results of family orientated therapy with schizophrenics were seen as comparing favourably with those reported for other methods of treatment (Esterson et al, 1965).

The four organisers of the Congress on The Dialectics of Liberation held in London in July 1967 were all identified by Cooper (1968) as anti-psychiatrists. Besides himself, these were R.D. Laing, Joseph Berke and Leon Redler. I want to consider the contributions of each of these people to anti-psychiatry, using them as examples of how it evolved.

Cooper (1967) also made reference to Thomas Szasz (1972) to support the critique of mental illness as a medical disease. Laing and Szasz are commonly seen as the most important representatives of anti-psychiatry, despite the rejection by both of them of the use of the term of themselves.

However, to combine unthinkingly the perspectives of these two authors does not do justice to their major disagreements. We will consider these differences later in the chapter when we discuss the work of Szasz. For the moment, I want to point out that in the origins of anti-psychiatry, Cooper did not apparently notice the differences between Szasz and the other anti-psychiatrists. He seems to have set the trend for neglecting and glossing over this conflict at the heart of anti-psychiatry.

Cooper may have been the first to use the designation 'anti-psychiatry', but some of the concepts that became incorporated into its thinking had been developed before the publication of his book. In particular, R.D. Laing had already published *The divided self* and *Self and others* and his study with Aaron Esterson on *Sanity, madness and the family*. We will turn next to the work of Laing.

R.D. Laing

The basic purpose of Laing's (1960) first book *The divided self* was to make madness, and the process of going mad, comprehensible. To do this, Laing resorted to the existential tradition in philosophy. He described the schizoid existence of persons split from the world and themselves. This way of being is based on anxiety due to ontological insecurity because of the lack of a strong sense of personal identity. This deficient sense of basic unity leads to the unembodied self, which experiences itself as detached from the body. The body, therefore, becomes felt as part of a false-self system. As far as Laing was concerned, and this may have been the reason for the success of the book, comparatively little had been written about the self that is divided in this way.

Transition to psychosis occurs when these defences fail in their primary purpose of keeping the self alive. The inner self loses any firmly anchored identity and if the veil of the false-self is removed, the individual expresses the 'existential' truth about him/herself in a psychotic matter-of-fact way.

Laing undertook research at the Tavistock Institute of Human Relations and the Tavistock Clinic on interactional processes, especially in marriages and families, with particular but not exclusive reference to psychosis. His second book *The self and others* (Laing, 1961) was part of the outcome of this research. It is a study of interpersonal relations. An understanding of how an individual acts on others and how others act on him/her is essential for an adequate account of the experience and behaviour of persons. Like Cooper, Laing mentions Bateson's double-bind theory as one way in which a person can be in a false and untenable position. He also shows he was influenced by the paper by Searles (1959) on 'The effort to drive the other person crazy'.

Sanity, madness and the family (Laing & Esterson, 1964) was the result of five years studying the families of schizophrenics. It is a phenomenological study in the sense that the judgement that the diagnosed patient is behaving in a biologically dysfunctional (hence pathological) way is held in parenthesis. The aim was to establish the social intelligibility of the events in the family that prompted the diagnosis of schizophrenia in one of its members. Unlike *The divided self* and *The self and others*, the case histories are allowed to stand for themselves with little elaboration of theory. Esterson (1972) later enriched the details of one of these families in *The leaves of spring*.

Laing (1967) in *The politics of experience* and *The bird of paradise* moved on to describe how humanity is estranged from its authentic possibilities. Schizophrenia is a special strategy that a person creates to live in an unliveable situation. It is a label applied to people as part of a psychiatric ceremonial. For some people, the schizophrenic process may be a natural healing process, but this is generally prevented from happening in our society.

The politics of experience provides a stark, political perspective that was absent from his earlier work. Laing acknowledged for the later Penguin edition of *The divided self* that, as far as he was concerned, he did not originally focus enough on social context when attempting to describe individual existence. He became explicit that civilisation represses transcendence and so-called 'normality' is too often an abdication of our true potentialities.

The politics of experience and *The bird of paradise* was first published by Penguin books. Most of the contents had been published as articles or lectures during 1964/5. *The divided self* was republished by Penguin in 1965 under the Pelican imprint, and Laing's other books were also eventually republished by Penguin making him a bestseller and cult figure. Laing helped to articulate for the counter-culture the need for the free spirit of the age to escape from the nightmare of the world (Nuttall, 1970).

In 1965 Laing and colleagues founded the Philadelphia Association (PA) as a charity. The PA leased Kingsley Hall, which was the first of several therapeutic community households that it established. Kingsley Hall did not attempt to 'cure' but provided a place where 'some may encounter selves long forgotten or distorted' (Schatzman, 1972). The local community was largely hostile to the project. Windows were regularly smashed, faeces pushed through the letter box and residents harassed at local shops. After five years, Kingsley Hall was largely trashed and uninhabitable. Even for Laing, Kingsley Hall was 'not a roaring success' (Mullan, 1995).

In March 1971, Laing went to Ceylon, where he spent two months studying meditation in a Buddhist retreat. In India he spent three weeks studying under Gangroti Baba, a Hindu ascetic, who initiated him into the cult of the Hindu goddess Kali. He also spent time learning Sanskrit and visiting Govinda Lama, who had been a guru to Timothy Leary and Richard Alpert. For many commentators, this retreat symbolised a lack of commitment to the theory and therapy of mainstream psychiatry (Sedgwick, 1972).

Laing returned the following year and lectured to large audiences as well as engaging in private practice. *Knots* (Laing, 1970) was another bestseller. It described relational 'knots' or in Laing's words 'tangles, fankles, impasses, disjunctions, whirligogs, binds'. It was couched in playful, poetic language and was successfully performed on stage.

The politics of the family (Laing, 1971) reinforced the importance of understanding people in social situations. Laing made clear that he was not asserting that families cause schizophrenia. Despite this clear statement, the charge has been repeatedly made. For example, Clare (1997a) states:

> Many parents of sufferers from schizophrenia cannot forgive him [Laing] ... for adding the guilt of having 'caused' the illness in the first place to their strains and stresses of having to be the main providers of support.

Even if it is true that many parents cannot forgive him, it is obviously wrong and naïve to suggest that he was blaming families. Laing was not talking about conscious, deliberate motivation to cause harm.

The facts of life (Laing, 1976) was a somewhat disjointed book which was not a bestseller. The style included poetic discourse and there was little attempt to provide an overarching theoretical perspective. As Laing himself said, 'What is here are sketches of my childhood, first questions, speculations, observations, reflections on conception, intra-uterine life, being born and giving birth'. It seemed at least credible to him that prenatal patterns may be mapped onto natal and postnatal experience. Laing developed 'birthing' as a component of his practice following the technique of Elizabeth Fehr. He thought it more than likely that 'many of us are suffering lasting effects from our umbilical cords being cut too soon'.

Despite Laing's hopes, this book was not a success and its thematic inconsistencies may be said to have confirmed Sedgwick's (1972) prediction that there was little hope of further developments of Laing's psychiatric framework. As Laing himself said, 'I wanted to get into writing again but I couldn't' (Mullan, 1995). *Do you love me?* (Laing, 1977), *Conversations with children* (Laing, 1978) and *Sonnets* (Laing, 1979a) were similar attempts to express a certain sensibility. *Conversations with children* sold well in translation (Mullan, 1995).

The voice of experience (Laing, 1982) is on the whole better written and probably merits more serious consideration, as Laing himself claimed (Mullan, 1995). Laing discussed the relationship between experience and scientific fact. He reviewed the psychoanalytic literature on psychological life before birth. Laing's themes about intrauterine life are not always easy to follow and the book unfortunately still fails to provide a coherent account of this aspect of his work.

Laing's last published book was his memoir *Wisdom, madness and folly* (Laing, 1985). It reinforced how mainstream psychiatry tends to avoid the patient as a person. He repeated the disclaimer he had made several times previously about not being an anti-psychiatrist but conceded that he agreed with the anti-psychiatric thesis that 'by and large psychiatry functions to exclude and repress those elements society wants excluded and repressed'.

Laing's (1987) assessment of his own work can be found in an entry he wrote for *The Oxford companion to the mind*. He regarded his contribution as operating in a field that can be broadly defined as 'empirical interpersonal phenomenology', which is a branch of social phenomenology. Objective 'Galilean' natural science may not deal adequately with the uncertainty and enigmas of personal interaction. Laing, therefore, thought the main significance of his work may be 'what it discloses or reveals of a way of looking which enables what he [Laing] describes to be seen'.

David Cooper

After *Psychiatry and anti-psychiatry*, Cooper (1971) wrote *The death of the family*. He wanted liberation from the family, which he saw as an ideological conditioning device that reinforces the power of the ruling class in an exploitative society. A commune of people living closely together, either under the same roof or in a more diffused network, was seen as a potential alternative form of micro-social organisation. For Cooper, the meaning of revolution in the first world was a 'radical dissolution of false egoic structures in which one is brought up to experience oneself'. The urban guerrilla war may need to be fought with molatov cocktails, but spontaneous self-assertion of full personal autonomy should be seen in itself as a decisive act of counterviolence against the system.

As pointed out by Laing, Cooper's form of revolution was a 'surreal distillate' (Mullan, 1995). Cooper was a member of the South African Communist Party and was sent to Poland and China to be trained as a professional revolutionary. He never returned to South Africa because he was known by South African intelligence and was frightened he would be killed.

His next book, *The grammar of living*, made clear that Cooper (1974) was continuing his revolutionary work on self and society. He noted that some of the contents of the book were learnt during periods of incarceration. He viewed *The death of the family* as largely a revolt against first-world values, but *The grammar of living*, he thought, merited a rather cooler reception. The blurb on the front cover flap, however, warned that many would still find the book offensive and obscene. Cooper described the conditions for a good voyage on LSD. He argued for liberation of an orgasmic ecstasy and believed that initiation of young children into orgasmic experiences would become part of a full education. In principle he could not exclude sexual relations from therapy. Nor could he ever submit to the gross or subtle injunctions of bourgeois society, by which he meant essentially the classical Marxist conception of the 'bourgeoisie being the ruling class in a fully developed capitalist society that rules or rather misrules and exploits through its ownership of the means of production'.

In the book, Cooper (1974) made an attempt to define anti-psychiatry. He saw it as reversing the rules of the psychiatric game of labelling and then systematically destroying people by making them obedient robots. The roles of patient and professional in a commune may be abolished through reversal. With the right people, who have themselves been through profound regression, attentive non-interference may open up experience rather than close it down. To go back and relive our lives is natural and necessary and the society that prevents it must be terminated. The subversive nature of anti-psychiatry includes radical sexual liberation. The anti-psychiatrist must give up financial and family security and be prepared to enter his/her own madness, perhaps even to the point of social invalidation. Cooper never hid his zealous fanaticism.

The language of madness (Cooper, 1980) allowed the madman in Cooper to address the madmen in us 'in the hope that the former madman speaks clearly or loudly enough for the latter to hear'. He talked about the time when he was literally temporarily mad, deluded that extra-terrestrial beings, appointed from another region in the cosmos, were amongst us. He continued to express his view that madness is the 'destructuring of the alienated structures of existence and the restructuring of a less alienated way of being'. His theme of 'orgasmic politics' was repeated, not so much to emphasis biological aspects as did Willhelm Reich, but to see orgasm in revolutionary, political terms. As far as he was concerned, non-psychiatry was coming into being. By this he meant that ' "mad" behaviour is to be contained, incorporated in and diffused though the whole society as a subversive source of creativity, spontaneity, not "disease" '. This state of non-psychiatry without mental illness or psychiatry could only be reached in a transformed, genuinely socialist society.

Laing's comment on the work of Cooper is pertinent: 'I [Laing] never found anything that he [Cooper] wrote of any particular use to me; in fact, I found it a bit embarrassing' (Mullan, 1995). Although Laing & Cooper (1964) wrote an exposition together in English of Sartrean terms related to dialectical rationality, they were independent characters. Laing enjoyed Cooper's state of mind, but he repeatedly denied he was an 'anti-psychiatrist', hence distancing himself from Cooper's excesses. Esterson (1976), too, made clear that, as far as he was concerned, *Sanity, madness and the family* was not an anti-psychiatric text. In fact, he saw anti-psychiatry, by which he meant the writings of Cooper and probably also of Laing, to the extent that he went along with Cooper, as a movement that had done enormous damage to the struggle against coercive, traditional psychiatry.

Cooper's excursion into family, sexual and revolutionary politics could be said to detract from his criticism of psychiatry. However, this critique continued to underpin his writings and was restated in a speech entitled 'What is schizophrenia?' to the Japanese Congress of Neurology and Psychiatry in Tokyo, May 1975, published as an appendix to *The language of madness*. As far as Cooper was concerned, schizophrenia does not exist as a disease entity in the ordinary medico-nosological sense. However, madness does exist and deviant behaviour that becomes sufficiently incomprehensible becomes stigmatised as schizophrenia. Here Cooper seems to build on the standard notion of psychosis as 'un-understandable' (Jaspers, 1963), at least for the social process of identification of mental illness, even though he personally thinks it is misguided to pathologise such behaviour. Following Foucault (1967), Cooper saw madness as only excluded from society after the European renaissance, controlled on behalf of the new bourgeois state. Schizophrenia must be understood as interpersonal. It, therefore, has a semantic reality even if it does not exist as a nosological entity. It is also the label for a certain social role.

Joseph Berke

Joseph Berke is an American physician who came to the UK to work with R.D. Laing. Initially he spent time at Dingleton hospital in Scotland with Maxwell Jones. At Kingsley Hall, he was involved with Mary Barnes, who became a celebrated case of the potential for psychosis to be a state in which the self renews itself. The book *Mary Barnes. Two accounts of a journey through madness* (Barnes & Berke, 1971) describes, from the point of view of both authors, Mary's disintegration into infantile behaviour and her reintegration as a creative adult. Although Barnes was Berke's patient, Laing (1972) did use Mary Barnes as an example of the merits of regression.

Berke may not have made an original contribution to anti-psychiatry but his writings (such as *Butterfly man*, Berke 1977) reiterated its main themes. The purpose of *Butterfly man* was to demonstrate the potentially abusive nature of psychiatry and to consider alternative strategies. Berke noted that the mainstream psychoanalyst D.W. Winnicott seemed to support the thesis that regression and psychosis could be mechanisms of healing and re-adaptation.

After Kingsley Hall, Berke with Morton Schatzmann and others set up the Arbours Association (www.arbourscentre.org.uk). The Arbours Crisis Centre provides immediate and intensive psychotherapeutic support for individuals, couples or families threatened by sudden mental and social breakdown. Three resident therapists live at the centre. They are assisted by a resource group of psychiatrists, psychotherapists, psychologists, nurses, social workers and other professionals. People who come to live at the centre are the 'guests' of the resident therapists.

There have been changes at the centre over the years. Originally it was run by a small group who offered their services virtually for free. Now it is registered by the local authorities and funded by social services and health authorities in the NHS health and social care internal market. One of the main functions initially was to provide an alternative to the traditional psychiatric hospital, seen as repressive and damaging, whereas now the function is more to provide a specialised service based on the therapeutic community model enriched by intensive psychoanalytic psychotherapy (Forti, 2002).

Leon Redler and the Philadelphia Association

Leon Redler also came from the United States to work with Maxwell Jones at Dingleton hospital. He then moved to London to work at

Kingsley Hall. He is a practising psychotherapist and also a practitioner of the Alexander Technique, Hatha Yoga and Zen. Although he has not written any significant contribution to anti-psychiatry, he was an apologist for Laing (eg. Redler, 1976). Contact with Laing encouraged Redler's pursuit of Zen and Buddhism (Gans & Redler, 2001). Redler remained loyal to Laing when Laing eventually left the Philadelphia Association (PA). Part of the reason for the split was Laing's interest in birth and pre-birth experience. Redler became Chair from February 1997 to February 1999, the first to hold that position since it was vacated by Laing in 1981. He has been said to embody the tradition that Laing generated in setting up the PA (Gans & Redler, 2001).

From the beginning, the aim of the Philadelphia Association (www. philadelphia-association.co.uk) was to 'change the way the "facts" of "mental health" and "mental illness" are seen' (Cooper, 1994). It has fostered the development of several therapeutic community households in London. Its training courses, although psychoanalytically orientated, built on Laing's interests in social phenomenology and spiritual traditions.

The PA is now a member of the psychoanalytic and psychodynamic section of the United Kingdom Council for Psychotherapy (UKCP), as is the Arbours Association. Members of the PA households are encouraged to be in individual psychoanalytic psychotherapy. The cost of staying in the houses has been funded by housing benefit and the social housing maintenance grant, unlike the Arbours Association which charges a fee.

Thomas Szasz

Thomas Szasz has posted a summary statement and manifesto on the website dedicated to his life and work (Thomas S. Szasz Cybercenter for Liberty and Responsibility, 2004, www.szasz.com). This is made up of 6 points:

1 *'The myth of mental illness'*. As far as Szasz is concerned, disease is defined as a physical lesion. Hence using the term 'mental illness' is a logical and semantic error. The metaphor of mental illness is literalised by postulating it has a physical basis so that it can serve as a justification for psychiatric interventions and institutions.

2 *Separation of psychiatry and the state*. The state should not interfere with mental health practice, which ought to be an individual voluntary activity. Szasz was trained as a psychoanalyst and undertakes private work.

3 *Presumption of competence*. Categorisation as a mental patient should not be understood as diminishing legal competence.

4   *Abolition of involuntary mental hospitalisation.* Involuntary
    treatment is violence defined as beneficence. Detention should only
    take place under the criminal justice system.
5   *Abolition of the insanity defence.* 'Excusing a person of responsibility
    for an otherwise criminal act on the basis of inability to form
    conscious intent is an act of legal mercy masquerading as an act of
    medical science.'
6   'Americans are faced with the task of abolishing psychiatric slavery.'
    As is apparent, Szasz is not afraid of polemical statements.

Szasz has published many books since his original *The myth of mental
illness* (Szasz, 1972). These books reiterate the themes of the summary
manifesto. Alongside these issues, Szasz acknowledges that belief in
mental illness as a disease of the brain is a negation of the distinction
between persons as social beings and bodies as physical objects. As he
himself says, there is something positively bizarre about the modern,
reductionist denial of persons (Szasz, 2001). This is reflected in the
widespread acceptance of unproven claims of physical causes of mental
illness.

As noted earlier, both Cooper and Laing made positive reference to
Szasz. This may have been primarily in relation to his anti-reductionist
stance. It is clear from the transcript of recorded conversations that Laing
made with Bob Mullan (1995) in the two years before he died that Laing
was not concerned to work through his differences with Szasz. He was
surprised that he was not more of an ally.

Szasz (1976) wrote a scathing critique of anti-psychiatry in *The New
Review*. As he himself said, 'Because both the anti-psychiatrists [Laing
and colleagues] and I [Szasz] oppose certain aspects of psychiatry, our
views are combined and confused, and we are often identified as the
common enemies of all of psychiatry'. Let's try to disentangle these
perspectives.

Szasz is critical of what he sees as Laing's inconsistency. If there is no
disease, there should be nothing to treat but the Philadelphia Association,
for example, accepts residents into its communities. Szasz called the
Philadelphia Association 'Laing's attempt to set up his version of the
Menninger clinic'. Kingsley Hall, though, differs from the Menninger
clinic 'in much the same way that a flophouse differs from a first-class
hotel'. Szasz is opposed to involuntary hospitalisation, whereas, as Redler
(1976) confirmed in his letter in response to Szasz's article, 'most of us
[Laing and colleagues] agree that even involuntary hospitalisation has a
place'. For Szasz, it is 'cant' to suggest that the madman is sane and that
society is insane, if there is no 'sickness' from which one can make the
journey to 'health' via regression.

Laing (1979b) did 'get his own back' in a book review in the *New Statesmen*. He called the argument of Szasz's books a 'diatribe'. Laing made clear that in his view it is 'a perfectly decent activity to seek to cultivate competence in skilful means of helping people whose relations with themselves and others have become an occasion for wretchedness'. On the other hand, the implication of Szasz's position is that undeserving or bad, 'ill' people will 'simply be left to rot or be punished'. Szasz would view such a comment as a 'smear', because although from his point of view 'mental illness' should not be a factor determining whether criminals are imprisoned, he is not proposing prisoners should be treated inhumanely. Recently, Szasz (2004a) has again reiterated how he differs from Laing.

The ideological nature of Szasz's libertarian, free-market principles means that, as far as he is concerned, it is evident that individuals have free will and are responsible for their behaviour. As Laing said, there is little attempt to provide an in-depth analysis of the structures of power and knowledge in Szasz's perspective. Instead, Szasz focuses on what he sees as medicine's threat to human liberty. Medical killing in Nazi Germany is seen as an example of paternalistic state protection of incompetent individuals in the interests of health. Doctors did see sterilisation as a therapeutic intervention to alleviate individual suffering (Braslow, 1997). Szasz sees the modern therapeutic state as infused by the same paternalistic ideology, in particular in relation to involuntary hospitalisation and the insanity defence.

Psychiatry and its critics

Anti-psychiatry has perhaps been defined more by the reaction of mainstream psychiatry than the protagonists themselves. This is reflected in the disavowals of the term, as already mentioned several times in the previous chapter and in this chapter, by the people seen as its main exponents, such as Laing and Szasz.

Sir Martin Roth (1973), when he was the first president of the Royal College of Psychiatrists, identified an international movement against psychiatry that he regarded as 'anti-medical, anti-therapeutic, anti-institutional and anti-scientific'. Clearly mainstream psychiatry, using Roth as an example, felt on the defensive about anti-psychiatry. We will look at this aspect further when considering the response of psychiatry, particularly American psychiatry, to the critique of psychiatric diagnosis that arose out of social labelling theory. At this point, it may also be worth noting that Roth's wholesale portrayal of criticism of psychiatry as little less than an abdication of reason and humanity may better be understood as a clash of different paradigms about how to practice psychiatry (Ingleby, 2004). I want also to return to this theme when discussing the nature of the essence of anti-psychiatry in conclusion.

We have already noted the diversity of views collected together under the umbrella of anti-psychiatry, particularly the altercation between Laing and Szasz. Roth & Kroll (1976) elaborated the different groupings into four (see Figure 2.1).

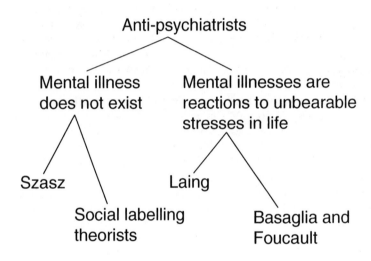

Figure 2.1 Subdivisions of Anti-psychiatry

The main dividing line is between those that argue that there is no such thing as mental illness, and those that say that mental illnesses are not diseases in the medical sense, but are reactions to unbearable stresses in life. This split is illustrated in the debate between Laing and Szasz. The first group can be further subdivided into those that state that mental illness does not exist in a primary sense, or in the words of Thomas Szasz (1972), who is the main proponent of this group, that 'mental illness is a myth'. The other subdivision would be those identified as social labelling theorists (eg. Thomas Scheff, 1999) who suggest that mental illness does not exist in the sense that it is merely the secondary consequence of identification by others in society. Further discussion about the social labelling perspective follows below.

The group who recognise that the use of the term mental illness is metaphorical and, thereby, do not want to minimise the suffering of people with mental health problems can also be subdivided into two. The first would include Laing, who emphasises that reactions identified as mental illness relate to interpersonal behaviour, particularly within the family. The second subdivision, containing authors like Franco Basaglia (Scheper-Hughes & Lovell, 1987) and Michel Foucault (1967), emphasise that broader societal factors rather than the family are involved in presentations of mental illness. Again, I want to look more closely at the contribution of Basaglia in the next section. Foucault's (1967) historical study of the conceptualisation of madness and, in particular, the isolation of madness in the great confinement in the madhouse in the 17th and 18th centuries, is included in anti-psychiatry because he views the reason of the Enlightenment as oppressive.

For reasons of space, this chapter cannot be comprehensive about the history of anti-psychiatry, and, in particular, cannot do justice to the international perspective noted by Roth (1973). For example, so-called French anti-psychiatry (Turkle, 2004) has been particularly identified with the work of Gilles Deleuze and Felix Guattari (1977). *Anti-oedipus* was these authors' provocative critique of discourses and institutions that repress desire. Another example would be Frantz Fanon (1967), who was head of the psychiatry department at the Blida-Joinville Hospital in Algeria in 1953, and later joined the Algerian National Liberation struggle, becoming a leader in the struggle against racism and for national liberation. Also worthy of mention, as noted in chapter 1, is the book *Not made of wood* by Jan Foudraine (1974). Foudraine could be seen as the Dutch counterpart of R.D. Laing.

Franco Basaglia and *Psichiatria Democratica*

Franco Basaglia worked at the University of Padua for 14 years before leaving to direct the asylum at Gorizia. There he was struck by the effects of institutionalisation (Basaglia, 1964), which Russell Barton (1959) had termed 'institutional neurosis'. He began his anti-institutional struggle to abolish the asylum. Paid work was introduced for patients to avoid exploitation. At the daily assemblea, everybody had a right to speak his or her mind. This forum became the place for expression of empowerment, collectivisation of responsibility and anti-institutional practice.

Initially Basaglia and other Gorizia colleagues came into contact with Maxwell Jones at Dingleton. Later on Basaglia became disillusioned with such reformist measures. As he understood it, the violence and exclusion that underlies social relations created a necessary political, class-related character to his fight. The asylum did not so much contain madness but rather poverty and misery. As expressed by his wife, with whom he worked closely, the asylum was 'a dumping ground for the under-privileged, a place of segregation and destruction where the real nature of social problems was concealed behind the alibi of psychiatric treatment and custody' (Basaglia, 1989).

Basaglia's (1967) first major work, *L'istituzione negata* (The institution denied) was widely circulated in Italy and abroad. It emphasised that what was required was a negation of the system: 'an institutional and scientific reversal that leads to the rejection of the therapeutic act as the resolution of social conflict'. The risk of defining the institution as a therapeutic community, as did Maxwell Jones, is that the oppositional nature of work in the mental health field is avoided.

Basaglia was influenced by the writings of Antonio Gramsci, a co-founder of the Italian Communist Party (Mollica, 1985) Health care workers, such as doctors, nurses and students, regarded as 'technicians of practical knowledge', were encouraged to contest their roles and recognise the social and political context of psychiatric problems. The ultimate refusal to be accomplices of the system may be seen in the mass resignation of the doctors at Gorizia because of failure to invest in community services.

Psichiatria Democratica was founded in 1973 and acted as a pressure group. In Italy, voluntary commitment procedures had been non-existent under the earlier 1904 law. The numbers of people in mental hospitals started to decline later than in the UK and USA. However, the population peak was still earlier (1963) than in some other European countries (Goodwin, 1997).

Law 180 was passed by the Italian parliament in May 1978. Basaglia was the principal architect of the new law. It prevented new admissions to existing mental hospitals and decreed a shift of perspective from segregation and control in the asylum to treatment and rehabilitation in society. A maximum of 15 beds was to be provided in Diagnosis and Treatment units in general hospitals.

Evaluation of the implementation of law 180 has been controversial (Ramon, 1989). The law was also a political compromise and could be said to have produced some inconsistencies. For example, locating the Diagnosis and Treatment Units in general hospitals ensures their medicalised character, which may be seen as undermining the 'anti-psychiatric' spirit of democratic psychiatry.

Basaglia worked in Parma from 1969-71 and moved to Trieste in 1971. The services in Trieste became the most important example of the success of democratic psychiatry. Franco Rotelli continued the work after Basaglia left in 1979 to take over psychiatric services in Rome. The first community structures began functioning in Trieste between 1975-77. A network of community mental health centres was eventually established, open 24 hours, with some attached beds, serving meals and providing domiciliary and walk-in services. Rehabilitation activities were developed: including training and recreational facilities; creative workshops; literacy and educational courses; and co-operatives that created jobs and enterprises that could compete on the open market.

Social labelling theory

The labelling perspective was intended largely as a critique of positivist theories of crime. It challenged the idea that there was a separate and distinct group of people who were intrinsically deviant, arguing instead that it was the reactions of others that defined acts as deviant and labelled those responsible (Becker, 1963). A further distinction was made between primary deviance, the initial rule-breaking act, and secondary deviance, the labelled person's response to the problems caused by the social reactions to their initial deviance (Lemert, 1967).

Scheff's (1999) book *Being mentally ill* is the best-known and most comprehensive application of labelling theory to mental illness. The theory proposes that a stereotyped notion of mental disorder becomes learnt in early childhood and is continually reaffirmed in ordinary social interaction and in the mass media. Labelled deviants may be rewarded by doctors and others for conforming to this idea of how an ill patient ought to behave and are systematically prevented from returning to the non-deviant role once the label has been applied. Labelling is, therefore, seen as an important cause of ongoing residual deviance. Initially, labelling was regarded as the single most important cause of careers of residual deviance but in later editions of the theory it is conceded that it is merely one of the most important causes.

Being mentally ill is of course not the only way of being deviant in society. The essential point of Scheff's theory is that the person recognised as mentally ill is the deviant for which society does not provide an explicit label. Labelling someone as mentally ill is defined by residual rule-breaking.

Scheff's theory is compatible with wider aspects of anti-psychiatry, such as the study of families of schizophrenics by Laing & Esterson (1964) in *Sanity, madness and the family*. For Scheff as much as for R.D. Laing, the label is a social event and the social event a political act.

Labelling theory has been challenged for several reasons. These include the relative neglect of 'primary deviance', the process of becoming deviant in the first place, and the said lack of evidence for the idea of a self-fulfilling prophecy or a career of deviancy. In particular, Gove (1980) has suggested that the evidence for labelling theory is so overwhelmingly negative that it should be abandoned. At the time that Gove first stated his criticisms, Scheff engaged with them combatively, but he now contents himself with pointing to such supporting evidence as Link & Cullen (1990) and admitting that the evidence for his theory is still sparse and mixed.

Although Scheff now recognises some excesses of his original theory, it did act as support for the view that mental illness is primarily of social origin. Scheff argues that the statement of a countertheory to the dominant biopsychiatric model, even if not totally valid, is worthwhile in itself. If only for this reason, his book became part of the identified corpus of anti-psychiatric writings.

The other study from a social labelling perspective that was seen as a major threat to mainstream psychiatry was by Rosenhan (1973) 'On being sane in insane places'. What Rosenhan did, in a classic study, was to arrange for his accomplices to be admitted to psychiatric hospital, each with a single complaint of hearing voices that said 'empty', 'hollow' or 'thud'. The auditory hallucinations were reported to be of three weeks duration and that they troubled the person greatly. Beyond alleging the symptoms and falsifying name, vocation and employment, no further alterations of person, history or circumstances were made. On admission to the psychiatric ward, each 'pseudopatient' stopped simulating any symptom of abnormality.

All pseudopatients received a psychiatric diagnosis: 11 were discharged with a diagnosis of schizophrenia, one with a diagnosis of manic-depressive psychosis. Eight of the pseudopatients were regarded as 'in remission', one as 'asymptomatic' and three as 'improved'. Length of hospitalisation ranged from 7 to 52 days, with an average of 19 days.

When the results of the study were met with disbelief, Rosenhan informed the staff of a research and teaching hospital that at some time during the following three months, one or more pseudopatients would attempt to be admitted. No such attempt was actually made. Yet approximately 10 per cent of 193 real patients were suspected by two or more staff members to be pseudopatients.

Rosenhan's conclusion was that professionals are unable to distinguish the sane from the insane. He maintained that psychiatric diagnosis is subjective and does not reflect inherent patient characteristics. As far as he was concerned, the pseudopatients had acquired a psychiatric label that sticks as a mark of inadequacy forever.

Robert Spitzer was chair of the Task Force that produced a major revision of the American Psychiatric Association's (1980) Diagnostic and Statistical Manual (DSM-III). Spitzer (1976) was also one of the main critics in the literature of Rosenhan's study and its conclusion. He was so panicked that psychiatric diagnoses may be unreliable that he made every effort to ensure that they were clearly defined (Spitzer & Fleiss, 1974). Although careful analysis of the evidence presented in reliability studies of psychiatric diagnosis may not be as negative as is commonly assumed, the commitment to increase diagnostic reliability became a goal in itself (Blashfield, 1984). Transparent rules were laid down for making each psychiatric diagnosis in DSM-III. The motivation for developing such operational criteria may have initially been to provide consistency in research (Feighner et al, 1972), but the attack from labelling theory reinforced the clinical need for reliable criteria.

This movement in classification has been called neo-Kraepelinian (Klerman, 1978), as it promotes many of the ideas of Emil Kraepelin, often regarded as the founder of modern psychiatry. It reinforced a scientific, biological perspective in psychiatry. The neo-Kraepelinian approach, and perhaps DSM-III in particular, provided a justification for mainstream psychiatry to re-establish the reality of mental illness, seen as under threat from labelling theory and anti-psychiatry in general. Such an approach has assumed an orthodox position in modern mental health practice and challenges to the biomedical model now tend to be dismissed as 'anti-psychiatry' (Double, 2002).

Against psychopathology

I want to make clear that although, in some ways, anti-psychiatry was merely a restatement of an interpretative paradigm of mental illness (Ingleby, 2004), its aspirations were not merely to replace the biomedical model with a biopsychological approach (see chapter 11). For example, David Cooper wrote:

> I'm certainly not going to argue a case for a social or socio-psychological aetiology of schizophrenia as opposed to an organic one, or as part of a complex aetiology involving all factors to a

varying extent. That would be a futile game if it were all centred on an 'entity' that did not exist in the first place.

Cooper, 1980: 154

Similarly, R.D. Laing, at times, may have quoted favourably from such psychologically-minded psychiatrists as Manfred Bleuler. However, there is a sense in which Laing wished to go a step further and to 'abandon the metaphor of pathology' (Mullan, 1995: 275). Or, as he also put it,

... all possible states of mind have to be regarded in the same way in order to diagnose any of them. Normal is as much a diagnosis as abnormal. The persistent, unremitting application of this one point of view year in and year out has its hazards for the psychiatrists.

Laing, 1982: 48

This abandonment of psychopathology is tied to acknowledgement of psychiatry as a social practice. The debate then becomes one about the social power and legitimacy of psychiatric practice. The close tie between social maladjustment and mental illness creates an unease that motivates anti-psychiatry, at least the Laingian version, to propose an alternative paradigm. Or, as Laing (1985) put it in his autobiography:

I began to dream of trying out a whole new approach without exclusion, segregation, seclusion, observation, control, repression, regimentation, excommunication, invalidation, hospitalization ... and so on: without those features of psychiatric practice that seemed to belong to the sphere of social power and structure rather than to medical therapeutics.

At times, this position created a dilemma for Laing, as he sought the endorsement of the psychiatric profession, demonstrated, for example, in his wish to be professor of psychiatry in Glasgow towards the end of his life (Mullan, 1995). For Berke and Redler, to different degrees, and essentially for Laing, the solution was to operate within psychotherapy, a voluntary practice outside the coercion of the Mental Health Act. Basgalia, by contrast, fully accepted the social nature of psychiatric practice within mental health law, stayed within it and altered it.

Relinquishing the notion of pathology may be seen as the essential feature of anti-psychiatry, as it is integral to the positions described in this chapter, albeit to varying degrees. It is what combines such opposing perspectives as those of Laing and Szasz. For example, Szasz suggests what is identified as 'mental illness' is better described as 'problems in living'. Laing and Szasz use different reasoning to arrive at the same conclusion about the invalidity of the notion of mental pathology.

If this rejection of psychopathology is what defines anti-psychiatry, it may be precisely in this area that anti-psychiatry could be said to have failed. Psychiatry is inevitably a social practice. The notion of mental illness is defined by psychological rather than physical dysfunction. (Farrell, 1979). Like Szasz, biomedical psychiatry identifies pathology with physical lesion. The error is to speculate beyond the evidence about the physical basis of mental dysfunction. Anti-psychiatry served a purpose in its critique of biomedical psychiatry, but may have gone too far in its abandonment of the notion of mental pathology altogether.

The essence of anti-psychiatry

In conclusion, I want to say a little more about what integrates the different anti-psychiatrists. The word 'anti-psychiatry' is not without meaning, but it does seem difficult to define precisely. Anti-psychiatry tends to be seen as a passing phase in the history of psychiatry (Tantam, 1991). In this sense it was an aberration, a discontinuity with the proper course of psychiatry. However, it is difficult to accept there was no value in the approach and what may be more beneficial is to look for the continuities, rather than discontinuities, with orthodox psychiatry (Gijswijt-Hofstra & Porter, 1998).

As discussed in the section on 'Psychiatry and its critics', what is clear is that mainstream psychiatry saw anti-psychiatry as a threat. This challenge to the biomedical hypothesis may be the uniting feature of anti-psychiatry. What is not so apparent is why this challenge needs to be seen as 'anti', 'other' and therefore outside psychiatry. After all, the biomedical approach is not the only model or paradigm in psychiatry. For example, the recent critique by Bentall (2003) utilises empirical, cognitive science. Bentall is a clinical psychologist and other mental health professionals may find it easier than psychiatrists to adopt an alternative to the biomedical model. However, although models of mental illness may be used to defend professional roles, they are not intrinsically tied to them. Bentall's book is an attack on mainstream psychiatric practice, and it arises not merely because of his professional allegiance.

Biopsychological and social approaches by psychiatrists themselves have not always been well articulated or appreciated for what they are. For example, the psychobiology of Adolf Meyer (Winters, 1951, 1952) is commonly criticised for its vague generalities (see chapter 10). Similarly, Arthur Kleinman's (1988) version of social psychiatry may be identified with cross-cultural psychiatry. Its implications, therefore, become restricted to that sphere rather than having a more general impact on mainstream psychiatry.

By contrast, anti-psychiatry stated its critique of biomedical psychiatry in a trenchant manner. As pointed out in the previous section, in fact it tended to go a step further in its opposition to the notion of psychopathology altogether. There was variation in this respect with, for example, some seeing the Italian reform as insufficiently radical because of its tendency to accept the possibility of organic aetiology of mental illness and its willingness to use psychotropic medication. Nonetheless, since the criticisms of anti-psychiatry were first stated, the nature of mental illness has tended to be subsumed under an 'anti-psychiatric' or a 'pro-psychiatric' position.

It seems essential to move beyond this polarisation. Whether this will be better expressed in relation to post-modernism and, in particular, a Foucauldian perspective (Bracken & Thomas, 2001, 2005) or a more pragmatic synthesis with psychosocial foundations (Double, 2002) remains to be seen.

Jones (1998) has suggested that objectification of the mentally ill makes psychiatry part of the problem rather than necessarily the solution to mental illness. This may be the essential feature of 'the "*anti*" element in anti-psychiatry'. This notion fits with the interests of the 'anti-psychiatrists' in the negative effects of institutionalisation in the asylums (Goffman, 1961). For example, both Berke and Redler came from the USA to work with Maxwell Jones at Dingleton. Basaglia was also initially interested in this work. Cooper and Laing experimented with therapeutic alternatives to avoid the objectifying nature of the psychiatric hospital. Anti-psychiatry became identified with the closure of the traditional asylum. A constructive outcome of 'anti-psychiatry' could be seen as the therapeutic communities of the Philadelphia Association and the Arbours Crisis Centre.

No doubt anti-psychiatry had its excesses. Ultimately Cooper, and possibly Laing, were more interested in seeking personal liberation than changing psychiatry. Few would want to go as far as Szasz in proposing running a society without specific mental health law. However, the term anti-psychiatry clearly covers more than these immoderate aspects. An historical analysis, of which this chapter is intended to be a part, should help to create a more reasonable evaluation of its merits.

3

From Anti-psychiatry to Critical Psychiatry

John M. Heaton

> There is a crack in everything.
> That's how the light gets in.
>
> Leonard Cohen Anthem

As described by Duncan Double in the previous chapter, the term 'anti-psychiatry' was coined in the 1960's probably by David Cooper in his books *Psychiatry and anti-psychiatry* (1967) and *The dialectics of liberation* (1968). Laing, Szasz and others were associated with it but many were uncomfortable with this label, notably Laing who rejected it (Mullan, 1995: 356). However it was a provocative title and for some years stuck to a motley group of critics of psychiatry. To David Cooper and some others it meant a psychiatrist who thought psychiatry had become a tool of capitalist imperialism; they were dedicated to creating a revolutionary role for psychiatric patients so that they would throw off their oppressors and be in the vanguard of a revolution. At the other extreme is Szasz, a libertarian whose primary value is personal responsibility. He argues that most contemporary psychiatry and psycho-analysis is based on an ideology of medical-therapeutic paternalism. He advocates that psychotherapy be recognised as a secular 'cure of souls' and that it be freed from state control and be recognised as a confidential, secular, and trustworthy setting for people, if they so wish, to look into their hearts and souls and, perhaps, make themselves better persons.

The trouble with the term 'anti-psychiatry' is that it is too general. As I have indicated it covers a wide spectrum of opposing political positions but it also is too general about a psychiatrist's job. Even a psychiatrist that gives electroconvulsive therapy (ECT), a technique that most anti-psychiatrists abhor, does more that give ECT all day long. Psychiatrists nowadays are mostly servants of the state and are responsible for arranging for places for disturbed people to stay, supervising the care of the increasing number of people suffering from some form of dementia and so on. Also a psychiatrist may investigate and diagnose physical disorders such as brain tumours presenting as psychiatric syndromes.

Another problem with the term 'anti-psychiatry' is that most of its adherents tended to make massive claims not merely against psychiatry but the social situation in which it is practised. Thus Cooper and many others blamed capitalism; Laing (1967: 108-19) blamed our secular world with its abdication from ecstasy and its mystification of experience; Szasz (1999) the ideology of medical-therapeutic paternalism. But psychiatrists can hardly be held to be entirely responsible for the society in which they practise and the subsequent demands made on them. Anti-psychiatrists themselves were obvious products of the very society that they blamed for the frequency of mental illness. They were part of an ideology common to America and Europe during the 1960s-70s which was not confined to psychiatry. Although they tended to put themselves in an authoritarian and exclusive position by taking a stand that appeared to be outside the society to which they belonged, they were part of a movement within it.

For these reasons I prefer the term 'critical psychiatry'. This has the advantage of being associated with the tradition of critical philosophy as practised by Socrates, the Greek sceptics, Kant and Wittgenstein. It is also continuous with R.D. Laing's 'provisional sceptical' strand of anti-psychiatry (Mullan, 1995: 310). These critiques spend a good deal of time analysing and condemning the incoherence and futility of their respective disciplines. Both emphasise the limits of science and scientific explanations and that our human form of life requires understanding our natural history.

Liberation

A frequent cry of anti-psychiatry is for liberation, perhaps best encapsulated in the famous 'Dialectics of Liberation' Conference organised in London in 1967 by David Cooper, Ronald Laing and others. The question of the nature of human freedom is very basic and there is a vast literature on it, which indicates that it is a subtle and vital question. It almost defines man, as we usually do not consider other mammals as free and responsible for their actions. We may free a tiger from a cage but this is negative freedom, freedom from the cage. But of course there is no such thing as complete independence either for tigers or for us; we are completely dependent on 'nature' for food, air, and so on as well as on our physiological processes.

Positive freedom is being 'free for or being open for'. Kant calls it the 'power' of man to 'determine himself from himself' (Kant, 1998: A534,

B562). Thus you can decide to go on reading this or to throw it away – you are responsible for whether you go on reading or not; if you are bored then you as well as I bear some responsibility for it. Freedom in this sense contrasts with causality. We cannot alter causal laws although we may alter their effects, as in the drug treatment of many diseases.

It is common in anti-psychiatry to understand freedom in negative terms. It is assumed that there is a basic human nature which is good, but that economic, social and historical forces have concealed and imprisoned it by some repressive mechanism. According to that hypothesis it would suffice to throw off or at least loosen these repressive chains so that humankind would become free to be herself and once again restore a full relationship to herself.

Acts of liberation may well be necessary: a colonial people may free itself from the coloniser; women may get to vote; gay people no longer be persecuted; the mentally ill be allowed to have more choice in what treatment they receive or whether they should have any 'treatment'. But no act of liberation is sufficient to establish the practice of freedom, as a knowledge of history shows us. The quest for freedom easily gets diverted into a series of illusory liberations from repression. Revolutions can result in an even greater tyranny than they replace: gay people, like heterosexuals, may be 'free' but deeply unhappy; we can talk 'freely' about sex and watch people on television having sex daily but whether our erotic, loving, passionate relationships are happier than before is doubtful.

Foucault (1981, 1988) has particularly insisted that the practice of liberty is more important than the repetitious affirmation that people, sexuality, and desire, must be set free; and the consequent claim by politicians, bureaucrats, and certain professionals that they can set them free. Is it obvious that by having one's desires liberated one will necessarily behave ethically and so pleasurably in relationships with others? We need to examine the ideas of domination and power and the role of others in the practice of our own freedom. Ethics is the deliberate form assumed by liberty.

Second nature

An important way that psychiatry can block the practice of liberty is by reducing human nature and experience to the purely natural scientific attempt to explain it. The natural scientific understanding of nature is a disenchanted conception of the natural world whose intelligibility is exhausted by causal laws. The mind is conceived as being wholly continuous with physical stimulations. Its cognitive capacities and abilities pick out entities that can be identified in a way that shows how they can be fitted into a single connected causal system. So all our beliefs, thoughts, feelings, experiences, etc. are ultimately part of a physical causal system. This leads to the belief that the brain is the cause of all our beliefs and feelings. So it seems reasonable enough to treat what a lay person would call a disorder of the mind, or perhaps person, as 'really' a disorder of the brain. Hence the therapeutic use of drugs, psychosurgery and other physical methods as fundamental in the treatment of psychosis and neurosis.

There is a huge literature criticising this picture which I cannot attempt to summarise. I mention McDowell's book *Mind and World* as it is a recent work and has been much commented on (Smith, 2002; Alweiss, 2000). He recaptures the Aristotelian idea that the normal mature human being is a rational animal, that is, our rationality is part of our animal nature but becomes our second nature.

The conception of the natural provided by the natural sciences is a realm of law; that is, the sciences try to explain the phenomena in the world in terms of laws, especially causal laws. So nature becomes a thing wholly apart from human activity and meaning. Thus the laws of the physiology and biochemistry of our brains are wholly apart from us, we cannot disobey them and most of us know little about them. Of course we can alter some of the functions of the brain by means of drugs but these too act purely causally. I cannot alter the serotonin level in my brain directly in the way that I can decide to raise my arm; although of course a suitable drug would alter it.

Our second nature is the realm of reason, decision, enjoyment, and freedom. Neurophysiologists tell us facts about the brain but it is equally a fact that I can decide to raise or lower my arm, give reasons why I changed my mind about where to go on holiday, be blamed for various faults in this chapter, enjoy watching a sunset, and so on. The notion of second nature enables us to understand these facts. These are legitimate forms of knowledge and experience that are not further translatable into the causal laws of science. Instead of a belief that flatly imposes human meaning onto the meaningless natural world, the notion of our second nature can be shown to be not reducible to or derivable from law governed nature, but nevertheless it is natural as it is the way we humans come to experience, negotiate, and shape our world.

Our second nature is the way it is because of the potentialities we are born with but crucially because of our upbringing. A chimpanzee brought up like a human infant does not develop a human second nature – it cannot learn a mother tongue which has the potentialities ours has. A human infant that has no connection with other humans – say it is brought up by wolves – cannot develop a human second nature unless rescued when it is still a child. The rich experience of human nature of the mature adult depends on her potentiality and her upbringing, the structure of her brain and how she has been brought up.

It is our up-bringing that moulds our second nature and initiates us into a culture and enables us to develop conceptual capacities which include a honed responsiveness to other human beings. This up-bringing at first is an initiation, as parents do not teach the child its mother tongue. Rather they respond appropriately to its stage of development and are part of an already constituted culture with a long history and orientation to the world. It is only a fairly mature child that can ask questions and have a concept of language.

A critical element of our second nature is the notion of freedom. The concept of freedom does not apply to the processes studied by the natural sciences. Biochemical processes do not choose but are explained in terms of causal laws. But our second nature is intimately concerned with freedom and spontaneity because it is partly constituted by rules we can choose to obey or disobey; we can be held responsible or asked to account for the way we follow or refuse to follow certain rules. We can act spontaneously in rule following, or feel that some rules are a burden and limit our freedom. Thus we can enjoy a game of chess, which has many rules, but feel the rules of taxation are a burden. Our notions of the norms of reason and the structures within which meaning comes into view are all part of our second nature as is our ability to create the natural sciences. Both the neurophysiologist and the schizophrenic have a basic nature describable in causal terms and a second nature.

One of the interesting points of psychiatry is that it spans the two natures of human beings. It is concerned with some disorders of the brain and sometimes other parts of the body where the laws of causality reign. But it is also concerned with our second nature because our initiation into it may be far from perfect. Our second nature develops best when we are loved, or at least respected, by those responsible for our initiation into culture. This often does not happen with resulting conflict and confusions. Psychotherapy is an attempt to clarify these.

But psychiatrists find it difficult to live with duality. So either our second nature is ignored and all disorder is explained in terms of brain processes. Or an extreme idealism is embraced, as in much psychoanalysis, where all disorders are explained as being at root caused by unconscious mental processes. It is one of the tasks of critical psychiatry to clarify the differences in specific cases, to differentiate and respect those conditions where there is a failure of causal mechanisms from those where there have been failures in the initiation and development of second nature.

Kant gave a vivid description of the response of our second nature:

> Suppose someone asserts of his lustful inclination that, when the desired object and the opportunity are present, it is quite irresistible to him; ask him whether, if a gallows were erected in front of the house where he finds this opportunity and he would be hanged on it immediately after gratifying his lust, he would not then control his inclination. One need not conjecture very long what he would reply.
>
> Kant, 1997: 27

Brain processes are determined by causal mechanisms and according to psychoanalysis mental processes are equally determined by unconscious forces. The person 'can't help it'. Kant's example shows, however, that our second nature enables us to make decisions, the man who would decide not to indulge his lusts under these circumstances is not equally a causal mechanism.

An urgent task for critical psychiatry is to attend to the practice of liberty and respect its place in our natural history, as most of the problems met by psychiatrists are those of our second nature.

Parrhesia

There were some fundamental texts that were vital to the thinking of David Cooper, Laing, and myself, which we often discussed. Sartre's *Transcendence of the ego,* the writings of Dionysius the Areopagite, Kierkegaard's *The sickness unto death,* some Buddhist texts, and for me Wittgenstein's *Tractatus* were amongst them. These texts are difficult and cannot be understood discursively in a few readings. They are not informative as is the literature of psychoanalysis and psychiatry. But this is their importance for critical psychiatry. For they are not geared towards any manifest content that one can grasp and communicate as truths which can become dogma. Their insights can only be rediscovered from one's own standpoint; one has to think through the gaps as they appear in the frustrations of reading them. It is the lines of force and intensity that need to come to light as they demand a transformative experience.

An important practice introduced by Laing was to have a copy of one or other of these texts in our community households – Merleau-Ponty and some Buddhist texts were the most popular. The point of this was not to turn people into amateur philosophers or Buddhists but to show that we are all 'in the same boat'. There is a long and distinguished tradition of thought about the human condition which is far greater than the narrow positivism of psychoanalysis and modern psychiatry and people were helped by becoming aware of it. Laing, I remember, was particularly fond of quoting from ancient texts, especially Buddhist and Christian ones, and would frequently use one or other of these texts in teaching psychotherapy students.

Sartre (1957) wrote of a pre-personal transcendental field producing the ego. Laing (1967) tried to give 'a feel' of 'it' in his chapters on the schizophrenic and transcendental experience and the ten day voyage. But mostly it has only been read as a description. Sartre's own words are relevant here: 'truth is action, my free act. Truth is not true if it is not lived and done' (Sartre, 1989). Perhaps some insight might be gained from discussing *parrhesia*.

This is the word used by Foucault to focus his thought on the practice of freedom (Foucault, 1988, 2001). It is an ancient Greek word and is translated as 'free speech' and was much discussed by the ancient Greek dramatists and philosophers. The *parrhesiastes* is someone who opens his heart and mind completely through his discourse, so he is truthful about what he thinks and feels. *Parrhesia* refers to the relationship between the speaker and what he says. Someone may report a lot of truths – she might rattle off truths about the anatomy and physiology of the brain but she is not necessarily practising *parrhesia*. She may be concerned to show off, to pass an exam, to act professionally and so on. Her relationship to the truths that she states is not her concern; she reports truths but is not truthful. The *parrhesiastes* avoids rhetorical devices which may influence her mind or the minds of her audience but which at the same time comes between them. Instead she expresses herself as directly as possible.

There are two types of *parrhesia* which were distinguished. There is the pejorative type which refers to the endless babbler whose 'chattering' consists in saying everything he has in mind without qualification, who was especially criticised by Plato as being stupid and potentially dangerous (Foucault, 2001: 13). Then there is the positive type which is to tell the truth of what one thinks; this involves a risk as she exposes herself to the person to whom she speaks who may become angry, shocked, sneering, patronising, etc. and so may obtain power over her. It involves political freedom, as under a tyranny it may be fatal to state frankly what one thinks to anyone.

Socrates developed the practice of *parrhesia* as a way of developing the proper care of the self (Foucault, 2001: 91-107) – it was a way of transforming the soul. The listener is provoked by the Socratic *logos* to speak of himself. This did not involve a confessional autobiography – this was developed later by Christianity – nor did it involve a narrative of the historical events in his life, but rather he had to show the relation between his rational discourse, the *logos*, and the way he lived; whether there was a true concord between his words and deeds. It was not individual arguments rather particular people and the aspects of their life and personality which made them respond as they did, that Socrates examined. So the uniqueness of each and the resulting interaction was respected.

The sophist can give fine and clever speeches, say on courage, but is not courageous himself. He does not take proper care of himself, although he may think he does and usually has plenty to say about how others should care for themselves. Philosophers have tended to develop a timeless, acontextual notion of reason that ignores its own values, interests, and origins. They tend to lecture, assuming an ahistorical reason that unifies multiplicities which the lecturer assumes he knows. Thus they ignore the unique relationship of each person to truth. As Laing (1967: 39-48) pointed out the metapsychology developed by Freud and his followers does the same. It has no category of 'I' and 'you'. How two mental apparatuses can relate to each other is unexamined. It is persons not apparatuses that can express themselves truthfully.

Socrates acted as a touchstone for people's way of life because he spoke freely and people recognised that what he said was in accord with what he thought and what he thought was visible in his actions. He practised freedom. He did not claim to have any special knowledge or qualification given by some authority. He did not speak according to the dictates of a theory. Truth does not come in the form of a prepared speech. It 'comes out' under its own power; it is artless as if one could speak it not by design or intention but truthfully. It makes no claim for the truth of what it says, there is no guarantor of truth outside of the truth telling. It is the relationship between two human beings which discloses the kind of relation they have to truth. This enables them to choose the kind of life that would be in accord with *logos,* ie. with courage, justice, and truthfulness, so that they would take proper care of themselves and others.

One of the difficulties Foucault discusses is how to recognise a *parrhesiastes*, a genuine truth-teller (Foucault, 2001: 134-42). This is a matter of great difficulty because our own self-love stands in the way – we are our own flatterers. Because of this we are not interested in recognising a *parrhesiastes* – we simply want to bask in flattery. Foucault, following Plutarch and Galen, suggests two criteria. First, there is conformity between what the real truth-teller says with how he behaves. Second, there is steadiness of mind. A person involved in self-flattery tends to be suggestible and so easily moved by the opinions and feelings of those around him, he tends to gravitate towards the powerful as he feels he can imbibe their power.

Galen, the great physician at the end of the second century, in his essay 'The diagnosis and cure of the soul's passions', after stating that self-love is the root of self-delusion tells us how to recognise someone who might cure us:

> When a man does not greet the powerful and wealthy by name, when he does not visit them, when he does not dine with them, when he lives a disciplined life, expect that man to speak the truth; try to come to a deeper knowledge of what kind of man he is (and this comes by long association).
>
> Quoted in Foucault, 2001: 140

In this path of knowing oneself it is important to see that what is at stake is the relation of oneself to truth. If this is so then this truth is not primarily theoretical; it does not depend on a model of the mind. Rather, as Foucault points out, the problem of memory is at the heart of it (Foucault, 2001: 166) – we need reminding rather than constructing models. For to the extent that we are involved in self-love we forget our relation between what we say and how we act – we remain enthralled by images. We need to remind ourselves or be reminded of what we have done and thought and so see the lack of harmony between them.

There are two sides to truth. One side is to determine whether our reasoning is correct and the evidence for our beliefs, this is the side that chiefly concerns the sciences. The other side is concerned with our relationship with the truth, the importance of being truthful, the relationship between truth telling and power. It is this that should be a central concern of critical psychiatry, for most people who seek psychiatric help are in various states of illusion or delusion, their relationship to the truth is disordered.

Psychotherapy

It is instructive to compare the practice of *parrhesia* with psychotherapy. I will mostly discuss Freud as he is by far the most influential psychotherapist in the last 100 years. The rule of free association is fundamental to psychoanalytic technique. This appears similar to *parrhesia* in that in both one is required to say freely what one thinks and feels, selecting nothing. Similarly Freud's insight into the importance of slips of the tongue and dreams in understanding mental conflict is relevant to the practice of *parrhesia*. For in both slips of the tongue and dreams we reveal that we have a disturbed relation to truth, we say or think or dream one thing yet our actions are not in harmony with it.

But there are radical differences. Psychoanalysis is a technique dependent on theoretical structures with which to measure, contain and control human behaviour – it is an exercise of power. The patient is conceived as an object and told to obey the rule of free association. As it is a rule that is often broken much of the treatment is concerned with explaining these breaks in order to control the patient. It is a rule given by the analyst who remains as anonymous as possible so his power is disguised and not questioned; if the patient does question it then his behaviour is interpreted as having an unconscious motive and so he is brought into line.

In the practice of *parrhesia* on the other hand, no rule is imposed and there is no place for anonymity. For the *parrhesiastes* does not think that the problem in neurosis is a causal one requiring an expert knowledge of mental mechanisms. Rather we are neurotic to the extent that we have lost touch with our reason and so are driven to fail to mean what we say. Slips of the tongue and dreams are a vivid example of this. Her job therefore is to be a touchstone for the other and so she must be recognised as a person who genuinely recognises and so practices freedom. It is vital that she is seen to be truthful and not merely believed to be because she has the right qualifications. Authentic power is developed in the struggle against forms of power that try to define human life in terms of facts rather than possibilities. Human beings, as beings who can lose themselves as well as find themselves, are the only beings for whom freedom is an issue. So freedom is always at stake in their living, it can never be a fact that is found once and for all.

To interpret slips of the tongue and dreams Freud created a structure, the psychical apparatus, to explain them in theoretical and causal terms; according to the rules of this structure they are determined by unconscious wishes. He took up the place of the anonymous expert, the one who knows. Now strict impartiality implies that one sees oneself from the outside and so can speak of oneself and the other in the same sense, objectively, as if they were reciprocal. It results in totalising oneself and the other and ignoring their singularity, what singles them outside the categories of the general and particular, their 'self-being' (Laing, 1961: 20).

Freud abstracted the mind from the activities of persons (Laing, 1967). He conceived it to be a discrete entity, a machine – the psychical apparatus – which is a purely determined mechanism. He thus could claim that the functions of the mind can be studied objectively like the functions of the liver or brain and so he could claim special expertise on it. Of course his method of study was different but essentially the patient's words and behaviour were the raw material for the analyst to observe and interpret. He thus separated a person's experience and actions from their ethical content and relation to freedom and so distorted the experience of dreaming, parapraxes and symptoms. As Foucault wrote:

> By breaking with the objectivity which fascinates waking consciousness and by reinstating the human subject in its radical freedom, the dream discloses paradoxically the movement of freedom toward the world, the point of origin from which freedom makes itself world.
>
> Foucault, 1993: 51

The *parrhesiastes* claims no special knowledge of the mind or language and does not abstract them from the activity of persons. She recognises that it is persons that forget, repress, dream, and so on, not minds or the unconscious, so understanding rather than explanations and theories are required. Therefore she recognises that it is not expert knowledge that is answerable to some theory and external authority that is needed but that it is the relation in which she and her patient stand to truthfulness that can disclose truth and so enable understanding to occur.

Freud did not think that the analyst's relation to the truth could be questioned. The analyst was a trained technician and so his qualifications were merely a matter for those who trained him. His interpretations and constructions must be correct as measured by psychoanalytic theory. But correctness is not the same as truth. Freud's qualification for founding this 'science' was his self-analysis – he never discussed this but as he was a 'genius', analysts rarely question it either, although they mostly believe that self-analysis for ordinary mortals is of doubtful value.

Freud defined the method of psychoanalysis in terms of anonymity, neutrality, confidentiality and the prohibition of personal relationships and his papers are written as if he followed this method. But in an analysis of forty-three cases seen by him it was found that he was never anonymous, was neutral 14 per cent of the time and violated confidentiality over 50 per cent of the time. His most important analysis was of his daughter Anna! His most successful cases were patients who idolised him and enabled him to confirm his theories and allowed him to triumph over his rivals Adler and Jung. Patients who openly raised questions about his theories were attacked by interpretations of their motives and as being resistant; usually they had a less successful outcome (Breger, 2000: 370). Clearly a positive response in both patient and Freud depended on what his patients did for him, whether they touched on his personal history, his need for flattery, his need for confirmation of his theories, and his need for high fees and if possible financial help to the cause of psychoanalysis. Nowhere was his or his patient's relationship to the truth questioned by him.

Freud claimed that he possessed the truth; thus he formed his famous Committee, a secret group of loyal followers who would protect the fundamental tenets of psychoanalysis – repression, the unconscious, and infantile sexuality. These tenets are now protected by the International Psychoanalytic Association. But there are fundamental differences between truth, belief and knowledge which are ignored by psychoanalysts and many psychotherapists. Beliefs and knowledge imply that there is a reality that is independent of them, after all many of our beliefs and much of our knowledge may be wrong. Both can be possessed but truth cannot. Thus my beliefs belong to me, of course many of them may be shared but some are probably exclusive to me, especially my beliefs about myself – I may believe I am a fine honest person but no one else may think so. Knowledge too can belong to one person or a small group. Suppose a group of people found a cheap way of turning lead to gold. They might well keep this knowledge to themselves and so possess it. But whether it was true or not that they could make gold would not belong to them, it is independent of them; thousands of chemists could check up on whether it was really gold that they made.

It is the same with psychoanalysis. Freud and most psychoanalysts claim that their method, beliefs and theories are essential to produce genuine mental health. Other therapies may produce improvement but it is only apparent as it is due to suggestion and so not true. This is an empirical statement but no clear evidence for it is brought. Psychoanalysts ignore the difficulty of enquiries into the nature of human desire and truth and their dependence on culture. They defend themselves from confronting them by theorising and invoking mechanisms of the mind such as projection which can be described theoretically but are not so easily recognised in action. So their beliefs become banal and reductive and are projected onto their patients. Conflicts become explicable in terms of well known motifs involving childhood, family problems, the Oedipus complex, castration and so on. The patient is subjected to the already-said and the already-thought. There is no place for her to say what has never been said: herself.

Freud's fundamental tenets were 'discovered' in his own analysis. But they were not discoveries of any reality independent of him, they were constructs or stories made up by him to make sense of his own confusions and those of his patients. His notion of the unconscious was no more than a heuristic principle which is assessed according to its usefulness in explaining certain clinical phenomena that interested him. Within his system and judging by his criteria he had good reason to believe in his 'discoveries'. But he never questioned the fixed background of his thoughts and that others might have very different values and forms of life. They were useful to him and to many others who have followed him but that does not mean they are universally true.

Truth is not audience relative – the truth of a statement has nothing to do with whether a given audience will be pleased to hear it or find it helpful in some way or believe it is correct (Williams, 2002: 165-71). This fundamental insight is not acknowledged by psychoanalysts as is illustrated by Kirsner (2000) in his study of psychoanalytic institutes. He studied the most important institutes in the US and showed that they have been largely riven by authoritarian cliques, power struggles and intrigues. This pattern is usual elsewhere. There is no attention to a concord between words and deeds. The psychoanalyst's impatience to 'know' and explain encourages conflict, acrimony and splits instead of free and respectful inquiry into the subtle field of human desire, the practice of freedom, and their relation to truth.

Kafka wrote:

> Psychology is impatience. All human errors are impatience, the premature breaking off of what is methodical, an apparent fencing in of the apparent thing.
>
> Kafka, 1991: 15

Cognitive therapy

Cognitive therapy has a very different history to psychoanalysis but it too claims to be scientific. Both depend on the notion that there are inner processes in the mind that act causally to produce memory, language use, beliefs and the like. In cognitive therapy these processes are explained in terms of the storing of representations that can play different functional roles. It is essential to this model that the mind is conceived as being essentially homogeneous; whether at the level of transducers, input systems, or central systems: 'all systems that perform nondemonstrative inferences, modular or otherwise, fall together as hypothesis projecting/confirming devices' (Fodor, 1983: 121). In other words cognitive therapy, like psychoanalysis, is a totalising system, its theory wipes out all differences between people and is concerned with minds rather than persons.

This picture of the mind has been criticised by Wittgenstein and those influenced by him (Heaton, 2000; Williams et al, 1999: esp. 240-59). This is not the place to state these criticisms in detail. Essentially he showed that understanding, belief, etc. do not make sense if they are assumed to occur in an isolated mind which is somehow separate from the body. There is no occurrent state of mind that constitutes meaning or believing. Rather they are states of a person *only within* a practice over time. Without the practice we can make no sense of understanding or belief, no matter what is supposed to be going on in a person's head.

The practice of truth-telling however respects the uniqueness of persons, their freedom and truth. It recognises that persons are embodies and live within a culture and that it is only within a culture that freedom, reason and truth make sense. So justice is not respected in people who think they can stand above others and explain them in terms of 'mind'.

The judgement whether someone is living a healthy life, truly caring for herself, is not up to a special professional group such as psychotherapists to decide. There are huge disagreements over what constitutes a healthy life, depending on our culture, religious beliefs, ethics and much else. Systems of psychotherapy develop knowledge but the truth of the system cannot depend on the therapists who know and believe in it but must depend on judgements independent of it.

There is no definition of truth – as has been proved by logicians such as Frege, Bertrand Russell, and Wittgenstein. It is an indefinable concept which if looked at too closely disappears (Williams, 2002: 63-83; Sluga, 2002). It is so basic to our understanding that it is impossible to reduce it to more primitive notions. So truth cannot belong to any system or group of people and that includes psychoanalysis. But that does not mean that it is mystical and untrustworthy. Rather it is a widely ramifying concept connected with notions of meaning, reference, correctness, belief, knowledge and so on. Interestingly in archaic languages such as ancient Greek there is no one word for truth, rather a variety of terms are used that imply truth and some that can be translated as 'true' (Williams, 2002: 271-7). But the relation between truth and truthfulness – which is related to fearless speech – was much closer then than it is now. For science and technology enable us to make lots of true statements but are not interested in our own relation to them.

Psychotherapists usually have no interest in their own or their patient's relation to truth. With an extraordinary lack of self reflection they assume that their knowledge of psychotherapy, transference, and the models of the mind on which these depend is necessarily truthful .A more reflective approach to the relationship between assertions of knowledge of the mind and what these assertions represent would reveal that it is impossible for any one person or school to 'have the truth' about psychotherapy. Human confusions and conflicts require genealogical understanding as they depend on the culture in which we are embedded and so it is impossible to stand completely outside them.

Genealogy

Genealogy is a term first used by Nietzsche to describe a critique of illusions – it has been developed by Foucault, Bernard Williams and many others. A good account of Nietzsche's concept of genealogy is in Deleuze (1983). Genealogy is a narrative that tries to make a cultural phenomenon intelligible by describing the way it came about. In contrast to the ordinary historian the genealogist traces patterns of descent from the present backward without seeking their formal beginnings. So he does not construct continuous narratives of the modifications that have lead to the present but rather his emphasis is on the erratic and discontinuous path of history. It is intended to serve the aims of naturalism, that is the significance of our non-genetic learning, our second nature and its relation to power and freedom. The relations between culture and psychology and between both of these and biology is its concern (Williams, 2002: 20-40). Its difficulty is that it holds up before the reader's lens a sign saying that something may be true and then tries to vacate the spot before the shutter clicks (Williams, 2002: 18-19). This is because the genealogist is aware that both he and his reader are part of the culture he is describing and she is reading. But no culture or member of it is static – they are subject to a multitude of forces many of which we do not understand or are even aware of.

Thus all human beings need to make and listen to music, it is part of our psychological make-up and so we can make generalities about it. But to understand the emergence of total chromaticism in the work of Schoenberg and others in the early 20th century in Europe requires a study of a particular human culture and the play of forces and values within it; as well as the genetic forces that enable human beings to create music whereas chimpanzees can only respond to rhythm and sounds. Genealogy tries to account for the actual existence of the historical reality it is exploring.

Genealogy is of great importance in understanding the problematic of 'pouvoir-savoir', power and knowledge in psychiatry as Foucault has shown (Foucault, 1967). It can show the way that psychiatry lets itself be driven by the various forces in culture to imagine that a state is objective when it is actually created by cultural forces of which most psychiatrists are unaware.

Take the contemporary problem of personality disorder in psychiatry. We are told that personality disorder is now a major public health problem. It affects a substantial proportion of the population and is a burden on health care, and the social and criminal justice agencies (Tyrer et al, 2003: 5). How has this problem arisen? Is there an objective condition of 'personality disorder' which requires identification, treatment, and prevention? Should we conceptualise it in the same way as we think of the treatment and prevention of a disease like typhoid?

Human beings have always had to find ways of 'dealing' with people they find difficult to get on with. Most societies have created laws to help with this problem. Thus there are laws prohibiting certain forms of violence and nuisance and most of us are aware of these laws, know who can enforce them and the punishment if we disobey them. Most societies do not look at the problem as a personality disorder, that is, a disorder confined to an individual.

Now there are big problems with the notion of personality disorder. It is admitted that it cannot be defined and there is little consensus regarding diagnostic instruments. For example is a terrorist suffering from a personality disorder? It depends on the political views of whoever is speaking. It is defined as 'an enduring pattern of inner experience and behaviour which is inflexible, pervasive, stable and of long duration', yet it is admitted that actually the 'condition' shows major fluctuations and major problems remain as to re-test reliability (Tyrer et al, 2003). The very concept of personality is controversial and there are many incompatible theories of it; it is unclear precisely what a theory of personality is supposed to achieve and the grounds on which a personality is judged to be normal or not. Thus are the grounds that of an ethical judgement or an empirical medical one? It is known that antisocial personality disorder is usually preceded by persistent conduct problems in childhood but this was known to Aristotle (Sherman, 1989) and most ancient thinkers. They concluded that the upbringing of children is very important not only for the child but also for society.

To the genealogist the question is how the concept of personality disorder has arisen in the last 100 years or so in Western societies so that it is now taken as an objective given. Of course a thorough answer would be a study in itself – I can only make a few remarks. In the late 19th and the early 20th centuries the success of science and technology was accompanied by a huge growth in professional experts such as probation officers, guidance counsellors, social workers, and psychoanalysts, whose primary job was to advise people on how to control their behaviour. This was marked not merely by rather modest developments in scholarly knowledge but by institutional positions that formalised such expertise and gave the experts a measure of bureaucratic authority. So the expertise was granted not only by what the expert knew, but also by the institutional position the expert held.

When public and personal authority is undermined paid experts emerge to fill the gaps. The decline of the family has been countered by the rise of child-care experts, of marriage by experts on relationships, and so on. Naturally none of these experts are interested in the decline of personal authority as that would undermine their position. Thus in the balmy days of psychoanalysis Freud, Klein, and many other analysts thought that all children should be psychoanalysed and they psychoanalysed their own children, so replacing the authority of parents by the 'science' of psychoanalysis.

In the last 20 years or so there has been an enormous increase in the number of experts in the management of individual psychology especially emotion (Furedi, 2004). To give one statistic, in 1980 there was no reference to 'self-esteem' in 300 UK newspapers. By 1990 the figure was 103. And by 2000 there was a staggering 3,328 references to it (Furedi, 2004: 2-4). A low level of self-esteem is associated with a huge range of problems from crime to teenage pregnancy. As self-esteem is such a vague concept pretty well anyone can be made to feel they have this diagnosis. This opens the way to seeking professional help who then exercise control by normalising the sick role, encouraging us to seek identity through a diagnosis, so promoting the virtue of dependence on professional authority.

It is assumed that this authority is obtained from science. But these 'professionals' mostly had little understanding of the epistemology underlying the practice of the natural sciences but they developed languages that seemed scientific to the naïve. Einstein, for example, who had a deep understanding of the nature of the natural sciences, rejected Freud's attempt to get a Nobel prize for science on the grounds that he was not a scientific thinker. Nevertheless these experts claimed to have special knowledge and this gave them power and the institutional position to exercise it. The traditional notion that a professional person had special obligations and so should exercise moral authority over what he did was suppressed.

These practitioners developed an objective stance and were spectators whose job was to evaluate others and then devise suitable actions to correct them. They looked on activities from a functional perspective. What is correct functioning on the basis of a recognised knowledge? Was an action useful or harmful? Did it strive towards pleasure or reality? Freud (1911) defined reality as what is useful. So they replaced the activities and decisions between persons by abstract forces that were supposed to cause them all. Notions such as libido, instincts, mental processes, neurological processes, replaced attention to real activities such as loving, hating, speaking, disobeying, deciding and dreaming. The language of disease replaced that of health and justice. Discourses that are identified with knowledge claims and institutions seen as powerful replaced the voice of suffering. The authority of the state and commerce replaced the moral authority of the traditional professional.

So now almost any human difficulty is subsumed in functional terms. Thus lack of interest in sex in a particular woman at a particular time is 'dysfunctional' and so we develop an epidemiology, diagnosis and treatment for it. Work has always created difficulties for some so we now have a specific disorder 'workplace stress'. We become blind to the mercilessness of 'doing good'. People who already feel helpless and in distress are excluded from their sense of freedom and responsibility. They are told that they do not even know their own mind! The cause of the trouble is in the brain or in the unconscious. Psychoanalysts feel free to use techniques on people, to operate on their minds, without asking their permission and clearly explaining what they intend to do. Thus commonly the analyst may say nothing and keeps an impassive face on being consulted – they are being 'impersonal' and doing good – or so they believe. This is a form of mystification (Laing, 1961: 122) that enables the analyst to 'interpret' their 'unconscious'. It as if the best way to evaluate the powers of a fish is by seeing how long it can live on dry land.

Justice obtains when we see some person being harmed by a third. It involves persons, power and freedom. It depends on the particular culture in which it is being exercised. Psychoanalysis and much psychiatry obliterate their being accountable to justice because they claim to be treating minds, brains, or behaviour rather than persons. If a surgeon operates on a part of the body then whether he performs the operation correctly or not is a technical matter to be judged by those who know. Of course he must obtain permission to do the operation thereby respecting the patient's freedom to decide. If he does not or is drunk or downright incompetent then justice can step in. But psychoanalysts and psychiatrists, by reducing treatment of people to treatment of their minds or brains, prevent any judgement as to whether the person is being treated justly or not, that is whether their freedom is being respected. By treating 'minds' or behaviour or even better 'the unconscious' they can claim that they are purely concerned with whether their technique is being applied correctly and that of course is not a matter of justice but of expert opinion – which is of course their own. So any judgement as to whether the treatment itself is just can be dismissed, provided they are a paid up member of their professional group and have obeyed its 'ethical' code. Justice and professional responsibility is reduced to the mere obedience of a code.

Our second nature enables us to be free agents in the world. So we need to see the world aright if we are going to live spontaneously in it. This involves the ability to judge whether things are so or not. A child has to learn to discriminate the false from the true, to structure his attention in appropriate ways. How this goes depends heavily on his parenting. This 'structuring' is prior to any sort of reasoning and theory because our understanding of reason rests on our natural reactions in learning to speak and act in the world. Thus we cannot teach a child to play or laugh for these activities depend on our second nature but we can teach it to play particular games or laugh at particular jokes. As Wittgenstein put it:

> Instinct comes first, reasoning second. Not until there is a language game are there reasons.
>
> Wittgenstein, 1980: 689

So any therapy for disorders in our second nature which is guided by theories is putting the cart before the horse. The concord between words and deeds is uncovered in the practice of freedom where free speech takes place between two human beings who can acknowledge one another.

4

Transcultural Mental Health Care: The Challenge to Positivist Psychiatry

David Ingleby

In this chapter, I will try and explain why I think there is an important overlap between 'critical psychiatry' and the movement to provide better mental health care for migrants and ethnic minorities, which I have been involved in since the beginning of the 1990s. My interest in this movement was partly motivated by personal experience: I had myself relocated from Britain to the Netherlands in 1982 and had learned at first hand how complex the processes can be which accompany migration. But in more 'objective' terms, it was also dawning on me that ethnicity, cultural diversity and globalisation were becoming the burning issues of our time.

In the Netherlands, a movement devoted to improving mental health service provision for migrants and ethnic minorities has existed since the end of the 1970s. This movement consisted of a network of highly dedicated individuals, many of whom were themselves migrants. A lot of the issues they discussed were very familiar to me from my involvement in the critical movement in psychiatry and psychology. This was despite the fact that issues of race and culture had, in fact, received very little attention during the 1960s and 1970s. The critical movement's preoccupations were largely confined to white, Western society: gender and class differences, for example, were high on the agenda, but topics such as the link between colonialism and psychiatry, or the Western bias of psychological knowledge, did not come to the fore until later (eg. Fernando, 1991).

In three important respects, the movement for transcultural mental health care showed a strong overlap with the earlier critical movement.

1 There was a similar emphasis on the *social context* of psychiatric problems. People rejected the notion that problems were purely

located inside people's heads and looked for the situations that could make the so-called 'symptoms' intelligible.

2   The question of *power relations* was central to both movements – both the power relations between professionals and clients, and the way in which mental health care could help or hinder the 'empowerment' of marginalised groups in society.

3   Lastly, both movements argued for *new paradigms*; not simply for adding a new topic to the mainstream agenda, but for fundamentally rethinking theories, research methods and approaches to treatment.

In what follows, I will explore each of these themes in turn.

Critical psychiatry

First, however, I should say a bit more about what I take 'critical psychiatry' to be. Although the collection I edited in 1980 under that title was – I think – the first book to use the term, I would make no claim to having invented it myself or to having provided an authoritative definition of it. For me, critical psychiatry is at best a 'fuzzy set' – a loose coalition of thinkers and actors whose ideas display certain family resemblances, but who are not united by a common credo or agenda. Perhaps the best way to explain what it means to me is in autobiographical terms: how I myself experienced it.

As a psychology student at Cambridge at the beginning of the 1960s, 'clinical' topics fascinated me the most, but after graduating I rejected the option of joining this profession. Clinical psychology seemed to me a rather closed world, dominated by a few conflicting dogmas such as behaviour therapy, family therapy and psychoanalysis. My first experience with psychiatry in practice had been vacation work as a nursing assistant in a 'therapeutic community' at Littlemore Hospital, Oxford. This was an intense and gripping experience.

At the time, the ideas of Maxwell Jones were being put into practice at Littlemore by a daring and original colleague of his named Ben Pomryn. The hospital formed a striking portrait of contemporary psychiatry, being architecturally divided into two wings known as the 'A side' and the 'B side'. The A side was a monument to classical, Kraepelinian psychiatry: heavily sedated patients shuffled along the endless corridors or lay motionless on their beds, under the watchful eyes of a hierarchy of uniformed professionals. By contrast, the B side was teeming with activity and emotion: group meetings several times a day encouraged patients and staff alike – there were no uniforms to mark the difference – to 'let it all hang out'. The ensuing shouts, screams and laughter wafted across to the classical psychiatrists on the A side, who shook their heads in disbelief and concluded that their colleagues had gone completely and utterly mad.

On the B side we regarded ourselves as the ultimate in progressive psychiatry, but we were amazed to learn that other schools of thought existed which regarded our work as positively reactionary. At Littlemore, the ultimate gesture of defiance against the established order was made by two long-term inmates who one day – horror of horrors! – copulated in full daylight *on the cricket pitch*. Not long afterwards, however, we received a visit from an inmate of David Cooper's 'Villa 21', who informed us that this act had not been revolutionary at all. Only copulation between a staff member and a patient could aspire to that status. Treating schizophrenics in newfangled ways was not revolutionary, either: the task was to abolish the concept of schizophrenia itself. My curiosity was aroused and I went on to read the writings of Cooper, Laing and the other 'anti-psychiatrists'. Later, I moved to London and made first-hand acquaintance with the anti-psychiatry movement. I realised that, leaving aside the questionable issue of sex between staff and patients, there was a whole new discourse about mental disorders in the making, in terms of which the A side and the B side at Littlemore were actually not as different from each other as I had imagined.

Even now, I find it hard to categorise the 'anti-psychiatry' movement or to define what it basically stood for. Some of its members had overtly political ambitions; others preached individual self-realisation; others still had their sights set on harmony with the cosmos. Some valued the helping professions and sought to develop their therapeutic skills; others dismissed the concept of therapy as absurd. Some were erudite, others totally unschooled; there were refugees – philosophers, writers and artists – who had fled from communist Eastern Europe or the United States military draft.

Around the crucial year 1968, the whole of academia became caught up in a wave of critical fervour and was engaged in vehement discussions about its presuppositions and its role in society. The central theme of the critics was that society is not a harmonious whole, but a power struggle, and the important question everybody had to ask themselves was 'whose side am I on?' If you weren't part of the solution, you were part of the problem.

In the second half of the 1970s, a lectureship at Cambridge University helped me considerably in deepening my understanding of the historical and political issues surrounding mental health care. Figures such as Roy Porter and Bob Young were working out a critical approach to the history of medicine and biology, and the students I taught, both in social and political sciences and in medicine, were enthusiastic and receptive. I eagerly accepted a proposal from Penguin Books for an edited volume on the topic of mental health, and in 1980 – after a long delay, due to a combination of my own inefficiency and the publisher's – *Critical psychiatry* saw the light of day. The title was anything but original; the 1970s saw the rise of critical anthropology, critical biology and even, for all I know, critical tree surgery. However, by 1980 the critical movement in Britain had pretty much ground to a halt. Mrs. Thatcher was at the helm, Ronald Reagan was poised to take over in the USA, the economic recession was deepening and 1968 was beginning to feel like a very long time ago. It came as no surprise that the book's sales remained low. Looking back, however, it seems to me that the book managed to present many of the themes that characterised the critical movement in mental health.

What exactly was this movement? Firstly, although Laing and Cooper managed to capture the role of standard-bearers for the critical movement, it was actually much broader and deeper than the 'anti-psychiatric' views that they propagated. In 1997 I had the good fortune to attend a conference on the post-war history of psychiatry in Britain and the Netherlands, organised by Marijke Gijswijt-Hofstra and the flamboyant, brilliant and now sadly missed Roy Porter (see Gijswijt-Hofstra & Porter, 1998). The research studies presented at that meeting confirmed my impression that anti-psychiatry had seized a disproportionate amount of attention and that the critical movement was not only much broader, but also to a considerable extent a part of psychiatry itself. For example, much of the resistance to biological reductionism in psychiatry originated in the 'mental hygiene' movement, whose followers succeeded after the Second World War in placing social factors firmly on the agenda (even though they shied away from asserting *direct* links between social conditions and mental disorders) (see chapter 10).

At the Amsterdam conference, historians such as Jonathan Andrews and Colin Jones argued that Laing had borrowed ideas from psychiatric colleagues without attribution and constructed 'a heavily contrastive version of his opponent', in which progressive and innovatory elements within mental health care were ignored. Instead, all attention was focused on Kraepelinian intramural psychiatry. Anti-psychiatry seemed to reject out of hand the possibility that biological factors might play *some* role in *some* conditions. The critique of intramural psychiatric care was one-sided and indiscriminate, and lent itself all too easily for misuse by policy makers looking for ways to justify closing the hospitals and turning psychiatric patients on to the street. In the crude and over-simplified version which activists often adopted, anti-psychiatry presented a challenge which the psychiatric establishment had little difficulty in dismissing. One could even argue (though I don't really have the heart to do so) that by creating a rift in the progressive forces within mental health care, anti-psychiatry ultimately strengthened classical psychiatry and made it easier for the Kraepelinians and their allies in the pharmaceutical industry to make their spectacular comeback at the end of the 20th century.

Main ingredients of the critical movement in mental health

If there is such a thing as critical psychiatry, what are its main features? As I have said above, theological arguments about what this movement 'really' is are a bit pointless: a movement is whatever its followers make of it. I can only describe the two themes that seem to me, from my own personal position, to be central.

Positivist versus interpretative approaches

Critical psychiatry is not so much directed against a biological approach to mental illness as against a one-sidedly *positivist* approach. Under 'positivism', I understand the programme of modelling the human sciences on the natural sciences. A positivistic approach to environmental factors, in which these factors are regarded as blind forces impinging on a passive subject, is no less objectionable than a biological approach.

This issue is related to a very fundamental distinction between modes of knowledge, that between explanation and understanding (often referred to by the German terms *erklären* and *verstehen*).

a   A *positivistic* approach looks for causal explanations of human behaviour (*erklären*), using the notions of cause and effect. It usually starts from observed correlations and the laws or regularities that can be abstracted from these.

b   An *interpretative* approach regards people as actors or subjects who actively interpret their own experience and who act in meaningful ways. Understanding people (*verstehen*) is a matter of finding out 'what they are up to' or 'what they are trying to say'. The starting-point of such an approach is the person's *subjective experience* (what they say and feel); the social context of action plays a crucial role in this approach

Having been fascinated for years by the pervasiveness of this split, I find it convincing to regard these two approaches as two components of the mentality that characterises European thinking since the Enlightenment. The positivist approach views people as *objects* and is linked to the drive to manipulate – to uncover the laws governing things and people, and to use this knowledge to bring them under control. The interpretative approach is concerned to *emancipate* – to help people explore and express their subjectivity.

Many of the criticisms directed against classical psychiatry have been aimed at its habit of using a positivistic approach when – according to the critics – an interpretative one would be more appropriate. The 'normalising' approaches which I reviewed in the first chapter of *Critical psychiatry* (Ingleby, 1980b) all have in common that they try to recover the 'intelligibility' of behaviour or experience deemed by classical psychiatry to be merely symptoms of illness. In adopting this strategy, the critics are really saying that emancipation is more important than control. This makes it clear that in the last resort, we are not concerned here with an argument about what is 'really' going on, but with a clash of *values*.

The defence of the positivist approach is of course familiar. An exclusively interpretative approach is based on a naïve, romantic notion of an entirely conscious and free unitary human subject. Moreover, control – for instance over disease – is often desirable; getting a brain disorder under control which causes a person to act or feel in ways that are a threat to themselves and/or others, deserves to be regarded as a form of emancipation. Mental illness is precisely the area in which an interpretative approach runs up against its own limits – for it is precisely when behaviour does *not* seem to be intelligible in ordinary human terms that the psychiatrist is called in.

Only a few proponents of a 'normalising' approach, such as Thomas Szasz, rejected the positivist approach out of hand. What most critics objected to in classical psychiatry was not that it *sometimes* used a positivistic approach, but that it *always* did so. For die-hard Kraepelinians, interpreting the 'human sense' of behaviour and experience was an intrinsically unscientific and untrustworthy activity. However, if you never allow yourself to look for intelligibility, you will never find it: you will end up failing to recognise the patient as a fellow human being. This was the core of the accusation that R.D. Laing levelled against classical psychiatry, and it is as valid now as when he made it. It is fundamentally misguided to think that *either* an exclusively positivist approach, *or* an exclusively interpretative one, could ever do justice to the complexity of real human beings. Whereas some aspects of a person's behaviour may have to do with a brain disorder, or the double Scotch they just consumed, many other aspects have to be understood in terms of their 'human sense'. All too often, however, we see that applying a psychiatric diagnosis has the effect of invalidating and marginalising *the person as a whole*. Just as in R.D. Laing's day, the most glaring examples of this occur in the case of schizophrenia. Patients and relatives of schizophrenics are routinely encouraged to regard the condition as an illness that totally robs the person who has it of their humanity. As a result, *everything* the patient does, feels or thinks is regarded as not making sense or, at best, suspect. In this way, the diagnosis becomes a self-fulfilling property; for in a world in which nobody takes you seriously, it is impossible to lead a human life.

Critical psychiatry, therefore, does not regard mental illness as a 'myth'; rather, it insists that an emphasis on biological determinants must never blind us to the possible human sense of people's behaviour and experience. This means *combining* positivist and interpretative approaches. An example of such a 'mixed discourse', in the view of the philosopher Paul Ricoeur, is psychoanalysis. In fact, psychiatrists in their daily work – like the rest of us – unavoidably use a mixture of positivist and interpretative strategies. The latter, however, are mostly implicit and unanalysed: they consist of the 'commonsense' interpretations which we continually use in order to negotiate social life (Ingleby, 1982).

The power of psychiatry and its role in society

The conflict between positivist and interpretative paradigms is a long-standing one that, as I said above, seems inherent to modern European thought. Among psychologists at the beginning of the 20th century, it was referred to as 'the crisis in psychology'. However, when the critical movement started questioning the social role of mental health interventions and the way psychiatrists exercised their power, it was introducing a relatively new theme into the mental health area.

The most obvious abuses, which the critical movement focused attention on, were the blatant infringements of human rights that occurred when psychiatric diagnoses were used to suppress behaviour which could be recognised as a valid form of dissent. The Soviet Union was notorious for submitting political dissidents to forced psychiatric treatment, including confinement, sedation and electroshock treatment. Such 'totalitarian' practices were roundly condemned as an abuse of power by Western psychiatric associations. However, critics of psychiatry in the West argued that many interventions that were accepted as routine also amounted, in fact, to a comparable abuse of power. The gist of the critique was that whereas mental health interventions are carried out in the guise of benevolence ('it's for your own good'), to a greater or lesser extent they serve other interests: those of the profession, for example, or (more generally) those of social groups which have a vested interest in maintaining the *status quo*.

Feminist authors attacked the tendency to interpret the implicit protest of a 'depressed' housewife against her role as a purely endogenous disorder, to be treated chemically or surgically. Classical, reductionist asylum psychiatry was most vulnerable to this type of criticism. However, even when the relationship between therapist and client is less authoritarian and 'top-down', subtle forms of pressure can be used to invalidate non-pathologising interpretations of behaviour. Kathy Davis (1986), in a classic paper on 'problem reformulation', showed how subtly clients in therapy could be persuaded to drop their own interpretation of their problems in terms of their social situation, in favour of the 'intrapsychic' explanation favoured by the therapist. Necessary to the success of this operation (also known as 'blaming the victim') is the systematic neglect of the meaningfulness of behaviour, and of the social context that is crucial to its understanding.

It was not only the misuse of power in *individual* cases that gave rise to criticism. When social, moral or political problems are redefined in terms of 'mental health', as has happened increasingly over the last 150 years, they are, as it were, removed from the public domain; mental health professionals becomes arbiters over whole areas of human life which were previously treated as matters of general concern. This shift of power has been referred to as 'medicalisation', 'psychologisation', or by Habermas (1987) as 'colonisation of the lifeworld'. Because such matters are now regarded as matters of professional expertise, they are removed from the sphere of lay discussion and become the province of specialists. Peter Conrad (1980) coined the term 'medicalisation of deviance' to cover this process.

For example, the contents of the DSM (American Psychiatric Association, 1952, 1968, 1980, 1987, 1994) are drawn up and ratified by panels of experts from the psychiatric profession. Diagnoses of mental disorder are supposed to be value-free, ie. independent of the particular social norms that the person making the diagnosis adheres to. Yet all diagnoses contain, of necessity, a large number of implicit value judgements (see chapter 5). The committees which draw up these categories and define their boundaries are, therefore, fixating and reifying social norms. The classic example of this is the case of homosexuality, which ceased to be classified as a disorder when the social climate in the United States became more accepting of it. But all psychiatric diagnoses require that a person's behaviour and experience be judged against norms concerning what is 'reasonable', 'understandable' or 'acceptable'. To deny that these norms exist, or to exaggerate the extent of consensus over them, is to ensure that the use of diagnoses as an instrument of social regulation goes unchallenged.

The fate of the critical movement after the 1970s

In terms of my own career, the publication of *Critical psychiatry* turned out to be 'a bridge too far': the emphasis in my work on critical approaches to mental health proved to be a stumbling block in my application for tenure at Cambridge University in 1980. The University did not further its reputation for objectivity and even-handedness when it appointed Sir Martin Roth – at the time president of the Royal College of Psychiatrists, and a vehement defender of classical psychiatry – to the committee which was to consider my application (see Sedgwick, 1981). In any case, the writing was on the wall: the era of Thatcher and Reagan ushered in a period of diminishing academic freedom and a vehement backlash against the social criticism of the 1960s and 1970s.

This backlash was clearly discernible in the field of mental health, as social approaches came increasingly under attack and classical approaches to diagnosis and treatment began a triumphant return to power. The notion that all mental disorders were essentially brain diseases became more widely accepted than ever before. Massive investment in research and public relations by drug companies ensured a comfortable place for the biomedical model as front-runner in the field: psychoactive medication moved 'up-market' and became a culturally accepted response to the stresses and strains of modern life. 'Talking treatments' came to be regarded as wasteful and inefficient. Against the background of continual reorganisations in the health services, psychiatrists edged their way back to the dominant position that they had enjoyed before the heyday of interdisciplinary approaches in the 1970s.

The steadily increasing financial squeezes of the 1980s and 1990s were another factor obliging mental health services to streamline and rationalise their procedures. Standardised, 'evidence-based' approaches were implemented and the DSM became the conceptual grid for mental health services in most Western countries, thus consolidating the hold of the Kraepelinian model. In principle, the present-day stress on 'evidence' is healthy – but in practice, the research paradigms used to evaluate theories and treatments tend to be positivistic ones drawn from the biomedical field. As a result, competing approaches are marginalised still further. Little attention is paid to individual differences, while minority groups tend to be excluded from clinical samples. Whatever does not lend itself easily to quantitative research, such as the effects of intensive, long-term therapies, is regarded as non-existent. In this way we have reached a situation in which mental health is dominated by a streamlined 'no-nonsense' approach, which many dissatisfied users and professionals regard as the biggest nonsense of all. Moreover, the tendency to 'medicalise' or 'psychologise' problems has become so widespread that even the *British Medical Journal* devoted a special issue to the dangers of unnecessary medicalisation (British Medical Journal, 2002).

As far as my own career was concerned, I was fortunate enough to be able to move to a chair in Developmental Psychology at Utrecht University in the Netherlands, where – to my relief – I discovered that the critical movement was still in full swing. Until 1990 my group and I were able to carry out a wide-ranging programme of research on the increasing social influence of psychiatry and other 'psy' disciplines. In its scope, this work went beyond the 'critical psychiatry' which I had previously been involved with. Moreover, I discovered that many of the ideas others and I had previously taken for granted were now regarded as misguided and outdated.

What was at stake here was the shift from a neo-Marxist approach to a poststructuralist one, and the central issue concerned the concept of power. The critical movement had talked about interests and raised the question 'whose side are you on?' It saw power fundamentally in terms of repression and attacked professional notions as 'ideology' – attempts to pull the wool over people's eyes. But according to the French 'post-Marxists' and their followers, who were chiefly inspired by the work of Michel Foucault, this way of looking at power was inappropriate and ineffective. It is the *discourse* of psychiatrists and psychologists that has power, not their profession; to the extent that this discourse is socially accepted, it structures the way in which people give sense to and live out their lives. The important kind of power in the modern state, in other words, is not repressive but *productive*. The 'psy' complex does not undermine people's interests; rather, it *defines* those interests. It does not distort reality, but constructs its own truth. The followers of Foucault, of course, were also active in Britain, and I soon discovered that in their view, books such as *Critical psychiatry* were not part of the solution at all, but part of the problem (see Adlam & Rose, 1981).

Much of my work in the 1980s (eg. Ingleby 1983, 1985) was devoted to trying to reconcile these conflicting frameworks with each other. The Netherlands provided an ideal setting in which to study the transition from a traditional society, in which many aspects of people's lives were governed by religious authorities, to a fully 'modern' one, in which the influence of 'psy' professionals was wide-reaching. Whereas in Britain and the USA, this transition took place gradually and almost imperceptibly from the end of the 19th century onwards, it did not take place in the Netherlands until the 1960s; and when it did take place, the effects were very visible. The oft-repeated cliché that psychology and psychiatry are 'religions' and mental health professionals 'priests' becomes, in this context, very meaningful. An important role in smoothing the transition from religious to psychological authority was played by figures such as Kees Trimbos, the Catholic psychiatrist who succeeded in explaining the ideals of the Mental Hygiene Movement (optimal adaptation and self-fulfilment) in terms that would be acceptable to the church authorities. According to Trimbos, good mental health was in no way incompatible with true religiosity; on the contrary, it was a *precondition* for it (Abma, 1981).

During the 1980s, my colleagues and I at Utrecht carried out studies of child protection agencies, youth work, family health care, infant care, magazines for parents, day nursery provision, and drug policy. This research showed, indeed, that the concept of 'repressive' power did not give much insight into these modern phenomena. Quite the contrary – many lay people experienced the replacement of religious discourses on the question 'how to live?' by psychological ones as a liberation. New concepts and attitudes were eagerly assimilated by the general public, a process which the sociologist Abraham de Swaan and his colleagues (Brinkgreve et al, 1979) dubbed 'proto-professionalisation'. Modern professionals acquired their power in far more subtle ways than the white-jacketed, authoritarian psychiatrists of old. Moreover, one could not view psychiatrists apart from the mental health system as a whole; and this system itself had to be seen as part of a larger 'psy' complex, involving many professions and many forms of influence.

By the beginning of the 1990s, however, the backlash against critical social research had reached Holland as well, and the group I had been working with was disbanded. Luckily, I soon found another way of carrying on critical work on the mental health services – via the topic of migrants, refugees and ethnic minorities. As I mentioned at the outset, my interest in migration was stimulated by my own experiences; I also came in contact with highly dedicated and inspired individuals who were working to improve provisions in the Netherlands for these groups. Although at first this 'interculturalisation'[1] movement seemed to me rather uncritical – many people in it seemed to assume that providing more mental health care was *by definition* a good thing – I gradually came to realise that many of the themes of 'critical psychiatry' had, consciously or unconsciously, been adopted by it. This is what I will now try to illustrate.

The movement for transcultural mental health care

The issue of culture and mental health has come to the fore in the last quarter century, both in relation to service provision in non-Western countries and in the context of multicultural (Western) societies. What factors account for this recent rise in interest?

Firstly, with the globalisation of the world economy, Western approaches to mental health are being exported to other areas of the world and are having to be adapted to local conditions. This is leading to more awareness of the cultural relativity of the concept of 'mental health'. Secondly, over the last 35 years the volume of global migration has doubled. One in 30 of the world's population is now a migrant and there is a strong chance that the mental health services available to them will have been developed for a population culturally different from their own. In Western European countries, 8-10 per cent of the population is of non-European origin; the problems of providing adequate service provision for this group cannot be ignored any longer.

But (secondly) numbers alone do not create a need for reform: attitudes to migration and cultural difference also play a crucial role. In this respect, we can distinguish three different ideological periods.

Colonialism

In the colonial era, 'race' was the key concept and a clear hierarchy was presupposed, with Northern European whites at the top. Psychiatric descriptions focused on bizarre or exotic phenomena and were constructed so as to highlight *differences* between races, non-whites being described as far closer to animals than whites. The one exception to this tendency was Kraepelin, whose aim was to show the universal validity of his theories; he, therefore, set out to look for similarities and not differences between races.

Assimilation

The excesses of the Nazi's during the Second World War gave racism a bad name (although it must never be forgotten that the belief in racial hierarchies was also deep-rooted in the USA and Britain). The war also hastened the break-up of the colonial system. In the post-war climate of economic expansion, social mobility was encouraged and more emphasis was placed on the influence of environmental factors than on genetic ones. 'Culture' replaced 'race' as a descriptor of diversity between and within populations. Rates of international migration increased.

However, policies continued to emphasise the importance of cultural homogeneity and the superiority of white, middle-class culture. Migrants were expected to assimilate and programmes were developed to remedy the 'cultural deprivation' of minorities. At the international level, the WHO adopted a universalistic approach to medical research and service provision, in which Western theories and practices were assumed to be applicable in all corners of the world. In this period, therefore, there is little pluralism to be found in psychiatric theory and practice. Mental health care remained the province of whites, and minorities were hardly to be found at any level – as practitioners, researchers, teachers, students or research subjects. Even as clients they tended to be under-represented.

Multiculturalism

In the 1970s, the shortcomings of monocultural assimilation policies became increasingly apparent. Migrants and ethnic minorities did not, by and large, assimilate to the dominant majority culture, but instead learned to value and defend their own culture. Monoculturalism did not create harmony but antagonism, because it placed large sectors of the population in the category of second-class citizens. Multicultural policies, based on the notion of *integration* rather than *assimilation*, were developed in which minority groups were encouraged to retain their cultural identity. Multicultural policies were first introduced in the traditional migration countries (Canada, the USA, Australia) during the 1970s and were adopted by some European countries (Britain, the Netherlands) in the 1980s. 'Cultural relativism' became more widely accepted, replacing the notion of Western supremacy. Even the WHO started applying anthropological insights and began to acknowledge the validity of non-Western medical systems. (It is no coincidence that the intellectual movement known as 'post-modernism' attracted many followers in this period.)

Clearly, it is only in a climate of 'multiculturalism' that efforts to improving services for minority populations can get off the ground. As long as notions of (Western) racial or cultural supremacy dominate, such efforts will be disapproved of. A policy of compulsory assimilation is diametrically opposed to the goal of adapting service provisions to the needs of minorities. The resurgence of monoculturalism in many Western countries during the past few years is therefore a grave threat to the 'interculturalisation' of health care. In Holland this has taken concrete form: the present government has discontinued subsidies for this activity, arguing that the responsibility for migrant health lies with the migrants themselves.

In what follows, I will outline various strands in the movement to improve mental health care for migrants and ethnic minorities.

Topics in transcultural mental health care

Remedying 'underconsumption' of care

One of the earliest arguments for paying special attention to mental health care for minorities was not, in essence, a 'critical' one at all: it was the observation that members of these groups were simply not coming for treatment. The problem was *inaccessibility:* information about the available services was not reaching minority users, or they were not being referred by their GP's. To the extent that these users had an image of the services available, it was a negative one.

At the most basic level, highlighting this problem does not reflect a critical attitude. One may be concerned about the fact that BBC television programmes are hard to receive in South Wales, but this does not make one critical of the programmes themselves. On the contrary, the assumption would appear to be that the more people watch the programmes, the better! That, indeed, seemed to be the attitude of some workers at the start of the 'interculturalisation' movement: the good news about mental health must be brought to all sectors of the community.

However, improving accessibility soon becomes a critical affair. What if it turns out that the reception of BBC programmes in South Wales is perfectly adequate, but people are simply not tuning in to them? This analogy makes it clear that accessibility cannot be improved as long as the *satisfaction* with services is low. Some of the negative images of mental health services among minorities may be misguided – such as the notion they are only there for the insane – but others are based on bitter experience. To a certain extent, information campaigns and folders printed in different languages can remove misunderstandings and ignorance, and thus reduce the threshold for seeking professional help: but as long as the help is experienced as inadequate, there will be resistance to using the services.

Focusing on the social and psychological problems of migrants

Another theme that was already present from the beginning of the 'interculturalisation' movement concerned the stresses to which migrants were exposed. Health care workers in the poorer areas of the large cities saw at first hand that the conditions in which many migrants were living were causing widespread physical ill-health and mental suffering. To start with, there were the problems of migration itself – the loss of one's familiar world, broken relationships, 'acculturation stress'; then there were the hardships caused by low socioeconomic status, bad housing and marginalisation; and lastly the hostility of the host society, which discriminates and marginalises.

To some extent these factors could be accommodated within the public health framework of 'risk factors' predisposing to 'disorders'. This of itself presented no real challenge to positivist psychiatry, except in the most reductionist biological forms. However, many within the 'interculturalisation' movement adopted a more radical argument: they claimed that the supposed symptoms of disorder were, in fact, understandable responses to a difficult situation. The movement laid a strong emphasis on 'normalising' approaches – on looking for the 'human sense' of behaviour instead of automatically ascribing it to a disorder. Adopting such approaches requires immersing oneself in the life-world of the people one is trying to understand, and a basic requirement of work with minority clients is a readiness to spend much time listening to their accounts of their lives – for their lives may be very different from those of the mental health professionals.

One area where 'normalising' approaches became particularly prominent was in the care of refugees and asylum seekers. Whereas the standard clinical approach to this group involved focusing on the post-traumatic disorders which harrowing experiences in the country of origin might have given rise to, more critical workers tried also to see problems in the context of *present* stresses: not only the well-known stresses which accompany migration as such, but the particular stresses – prolonged uncertainty about one's future, restriction of one's liberty – which are the lot of asylum seekers (see Ingleby, 2004). Many workers in this area realised that it was 'mopping up with the tap on' (to use a Dutch expression) to try to patch up people's psychological problems without drawing attention to the social injustices they were in large measure caused by. 'Advocacy' – action at a political level – became recognised as an essential component of mental health care for this group.

'Cultural sensitivity'

A third theme in the interculturalisation movement was the importance of allowing for cultural differences. The stresses in a person's life could not be understood properly without understanding the meaning of events in their own culture. What does it mean, for example, for a grown man to be dependent on his wife for money, and on his children for practical advice? The answer to that question will have a lot to do with where the family comes from. Nor can one understand behaviour in the consulting room, and the complaints people present with, without taking into account the cultural context. Treatment methods also have to recognise the cultural factor. This stress on specialised interpretative skills was entirely lacking from Kraepelinian psychiatry, and only after much lobbying was any attention paid to the issue in later editions of the DSM.

However, there are very different notions of 'cultural sensitivity' in circulation. The mildest version is not critical at all: it concerns only the way in which care is 'packaged', not the content of the care itself. According to this approach, health workers should be aware of the pitfalls in intercultural relationships and should learn a few additional communication skills, but their basic approach – give or take a bit of 'fine tuning' – is applicable to everybody.

Yet once cultural differences started to be taken seriously, the concept turned out to be something of a Trojan horse. Health workers started to encounter concepts which didn't simply translate between cultures, and patterns of behaviour and experience which weren't the same as those presupposed by Western models of diagnosis and treatment. In this way, the search for 'cultural sensitivity' led people to question the presuppositions of the methods they had been trained to use, and even to the idea that *the culture of mental health services themselves had to change.* An important role was played here by the disciplines of ethnopsychiatry (predominately developed in France and Germany) and transcultural psychiatry (more associated with the United States and Britain). Medical anthropology, too, has expanded dramatically during the past 25 years.

A caution needs to be sounded, however, about the emphasis on 'culture' which has come to dominate care for migrants. What has taken root in psychology and psychiatry is, unfortunately, a static, homogenous concept of culture that has long since been abandoned by anthropologists themselves. This has encouraged a 'cook-book' approach to inter-culturalisation: find out to which cultural category the client belongs and look up the responses which are appropriate. This, of course, does no justice to the complex, layered and dynamic nature of cultures – in particular, *migrant* cultures. Ethnopsychiatry and transcultural psychiatry, which both have their roots in the colonial era, tend to focus on the exotic practices sometimes found in the countries migrants come from. However, whether this knowledge can help us much in helping migrants from these countries is very much an open question. At worst, the assumption of a cultural 'gap' which has to be 'bridged' acts as an excuse, in the words of Rob van Dijk (1998), for shortcomings which have quite different origins.

The notion of 'matching' supply and demand

The Dutch 'interculturalisation' movement has always had to gain support by allying itself with other, more widely accepted goals and slogans which dominate health care policy from time to time. At the beginning of the 1980's, 'bringing care to the community' was on everybody's lips:

under this banner the campaign to improve the accessibility of services for ethnic minorities was conducted. Another useful theme was the prevention of marginalisation and exclusion (eg. the WHO's slogan for World Health Day in 2001: 'Stop exclusion – Dare to care'). 'Culturally sensitive care' was a successful catchword in the days when a political consensus existed on the need for multicultural policies. Today, the same concerns are formulated in terms of concepts drawn from the philosophy of 'managed care' – in particular, the notion of matching supply and demand and developing 'needs-driven' services.

In physical medicine, 'matching' means basically that patients should get the treatments they need rather than those which the service providers like to give. In mental health care, the term acquires an additional, deeper meaning: treatment should be *meaningful* to the client in terms of his or her own perceptions, for it is essential that clients actively participate in the process of getting better. The same issues arise at the global level. Exporting psychiatric services to non-Western countries cannot succeed if the services are not accepted and appreciated by the population of those countries.

This, of course, was one of the issues which was dear to the heart of the critical movement in psychiatry; in Italy, the movement called itself *Psychiatria Democratica*, to emphasise the right of users to have a say in the mental health services they were provided with. However, the majority populations of Western countries have shown less and less interest in voicing a standpoint on these matters. Instead, what we see in these countries is the enormous success of 'proto-professionalisation': the lay population has a seemingly insatiable capacity to absorb professional notions concerning health and to assimilate the goals, models and concepts which health professionals propagate. (This is a perfect example of what the Foucauldians refer to as 'productive power'.) As a result, alternative discourses on mental health are almost squeezed out of existence: professional ideology has become common sense. The 'psy' complex has created a population which largely conforms to its own assumptions, which has been variously referred to as the 'therapeutic state' (Kittrie) or the 'psychiatric society' (Castel).

So we see that the reason why migrants present such a challenge for the mental health system is precisely because they can bring in viewpoints and ideals which have *not* been shaped by Western professional notions. Their misgivings about mental health services go to the root of what makes these services 'modern' and 'Western', and brings taken-for-granted assumptions clearly into focus. After all, it is only when you have contact with people who are not like yourself that you can form a conception of what you are like.

The ideal of 'needs-driven' services goes hand in hand with the notion of 'user involvement' and a 'bottom-up' approach to policy development. The use of qualitative research methods, which aim at developing a *dialogue* with respondents instead of presenting them with a set of boxes to be ticked, is an essential part of encouraging user involvement. Standardised positivist methods assume, of course, standardised users, and in a multicultural society this assumption is clearly absurd.

In some ways, the discussion which results when users with divergent cultural backgrounds are given a voice is even deeper and more wide-ranging than the debates which the critical movement started in the 1960s and 1970s. This discussion is at the level of *paradigms*, not just the 'fine-tuning' of accepted approaches. It concerns, for example, the way in which Westerners have learned to categorise their problems as mental, social or physical, and the existence of virtually separate care systems based on these categories. Western professionals often complain that migrant patients 'somatise' and fail to show insight into the 'intrapsychic' nature of their problems: but we could just as well say that the real problems lie in the dualisms of mental versus physical, individual versus social which our mental health care system has institutionalised.

Conclusion

I hope I have succeeded in explaining why I see a great deal of overlap between the movement to 'interculturalise' mental health care, and the movement we loosely call 'critical psychiatry'. The 'interculturalisation' movement has reasserted the importance of the social context to an understanding of people's mental problems, and has criticised the unwarranted 'medicalisation' or 'pathologisation' of these problems. It has argued for more power-sharing between professionals and users and more willingness to listen to divergent voices and demands. Lastly, it has called for a 'paradigm shift' in order to loosen the increasingly monolithic grip of positivistic orthodoxy on care provisions and lay culture. I hope that this makes clear that the significance of transcultural mental health care goes far beyond service provision for a small group of users.

Note

1 The word 'interculturalisation' is not used, as far as I know, in the USA or Britain. It is a useful Dutch invention which refers to the adaptation of services (education, health care etc.) to the needs of a culturally diverse population.

Part II

The Prospect of Critical Psychiatry

5

The Limits of Biomedical Models of Distress

Lucy Johnstone

Psychiatric theory and practice is based upon a biomedical model – that is, an assumption that mental distress is best understood as a *medical illness*; a disease process which involves an alteration of biological structure and functioning. This fact is so obvious that it may seem as if it does not need stating. However, it is exactly this taken-for-granted status that makes it so important to draw out and examine the assumptions behind the model, which will otherwise remain implicit but will nevertheless shape every aspect of our approaches to those in distress.

This can be illustrated, at the most basic level, by our use of language. Language shapes the way we think, and hence the way we act. The vocabulary of psychiatry is 'illness, patient, prognosis, remission, treatment'. Having conceptualised the problem in these terms, it seems to follow naturally that interventions should consist of 'diagnosis, admission, medication, ECT' in the context of 'hospitals, clinics, wards' and administered by 'doctors, nurses'. With a different starting point – say, the assumption that we are dealing with 'problems of living' not 'illnesses' – all of the above would suddenly seem questionable rather than inevitable.

This, of course, is why critics of psychiatric practice, both professionals and service users, have developed an alternative vocabulary (Wallcraft, 2003). However, policy makers, the media, popular advice columns and many campaigning organisations are still using biomedical terms and concepts. The National Service Framework for Mental Health (Department of Health, 1998b) uses phrases such as 'One adult in six suffers from one or other form of mental illness ... one person in 250 will have a psychotic illness such as schizophrenia or bipolar affective disorder ... many of these patients have not been getting the treatment and

81

care that they need ... assessment and diagnosis, treatment, rehabilitation' and so on. A drug company-sponsored information sheet says: 'Schizophrenia is a brain disorder with characteristic signs and symptoms probably due to physical and biochemical abnormalities in the brain' (Orion Pharma, 1995). The current move to evidence-based practice is based on an uncritical acceptance of terms such as 'schizophrenia' as a valid basis for conducting treatment trials. And there is no shortage of celebrities eager to talk about the 'biochemical imbalances' that have led to their depression, alcoholism, compulsive rituals and so on.

Of course, this is all perfectly valid if, in fact, the biomedical model of mental distress does seem to fit. But is it true? Or, to ask the same question in its currently fashionable form, is it evidence-based?

I would like to examine this question under three main headings; (1) psychiatric diagnosis, and claims about both the (2) biochemical and the (3) genetic factors in mental distress. First, though, I want to be clear what I am doing in this critique. I am not simply disputing certain facts or findings, although that is a part of it. Rather, I am challenging the whole paradigm on which the biomedical model is based. This paradigm can be characterised as *positivist, reductionist* and *deterministic*. These characteristics make biomedical psychiatry not only inappropriate for the study of human beings, but even in its own terms, bad science.

A shorthand summary of the ***positivist approach*** in science is *treating people as if they were objects*; the particular way of thinking that underpins traditional scientific enquiry in the natural sciences, in which theories, based on objective facts and observations, are tested in order to come to an ever more complete knowledge about the laws of nature. While this has been fruitful in many areas, its usefulness as applied to human emotional distress is much more debatable. (The classic essay by Ingleby, 1980b has a detailed discussion of the issues.) It is ironic that while much modern scientific thinking has moved well beyond this rather simplistic model (see, for example, Zohar, 1991; Capra, 1997), a particularly primitive version still holds sway in the field it is least suited to, psychiatry.

The positivist approach does not have to be ***reductionist***, but nevertheless, biomedical psychiatry abounds with examples of what could be called the *nothing but* approach; the view that people are no more than the sum total of their biochemical or other physiological reactions. Complex phenomena are thus reduced to simple or simplistic terms. Professor Steven Rose, the eminent neuroscientist, has repeatedly challenged the idea that social and psychological phenomena can be reduced to such terms, and that this kind of explanation is somehow 'truer' than others (Rose 1998). We can look at any human experience, such as depression, at a number of different levels – cultural, social, psychological, biochemical, genetic and so on – and each type of explanation is valid in its context. But to seek to reduce the experience of depression to a statement about neurotransmitter activity is to commit a whole range of logical errors – with the result that 'bad science drives out good' (Rose 1998).

Determinism, one of the consequences of reductionism, can be summarised as the *can't help it* view; what you do or experience is an inevitable result of your biology. This is sometimes seen as a useful way of avoiding blame and guilt. ('I can't help drinking, I have a disease called alcoholism.') The other side of the coin is that at the same time it deprives people of agency and responsibility leading to 'the belief that ultimately we are not in charge of our destiny but merely "lumbering robots" ' (Rose, 1998).

In short, this is the human being as a (faulty) machine. The positivist, reductionist and deterministic approach to mental distress is vividly illustrated in the following newspaper extracts quoting well-known doctors:

Medical treatment restores the normal level of the transmitters and with this the patient's sense of contentment. These biochemical abnormalities in the brain can no more be altered by 'snapping out of it' ... than a diabetic can alter their blood sugar by not thinking about insulin and food.

Stuttaford, 1999

If you think of the brain as a computer, in the schizophrenic the wiring is 99 per cent correct but there is a fault ... Like the computer, most of the time it works OK, but if you stress it too much it crashes.

Murray, 1994

One might well object to such a view of human beings on philosophical, ethical or religious grounds; this is a point that I will return to. For the moment, I would like to examine such claims in their own terms, ie. judged in the light of the available evidence from the scientific approach from which their authority derives. Even on these grounds, I will argue, they fall very far short.

Psychiatric diagnosis

'Diagnosis is the Holy Grail of psychiatry and the key to its legitimation' (Kovel 1980: 86). There are many reasons why diagnosis is important. It provides, at least in theory, an indication of appropriate treatments, a basis for research, and a way for professionals to communicate with each other, not to mention information and relief for patients and relatives. It should, ideally, point towards aetiology and enable predictions to be made about prognosis. Beyond all of this, though, there is an even more important reason why psychiatry needs to be able to claim that it has a valid and reliable classification system, and that is because this is absolutely crucial to its status as a legitimate branch of science – in this case, medical science. As psychiatrist Michael Shepherd puts it, 'To discard classification is to discard scientific thinking' (Shepherd 1976: 3). If there is no agreement on basic classification, then there is no basis for drawing up the general laws that constitute a body of scientific knowledge.

The implications are profound: if classification can be shown to be neither reliable nor valid, then everything that follows from the biomedical assumptions outlined above, our current interventions, settings, professionals, up to and including the language we use, would need fundamental revision.   Hence the statement 'The critique of diagnosis *is* the critique of psychiatry ... Diagnosis locates the parameters of normality and abnormality, demarcates the professional and institutional boundaries of the mental health system, and authorises psychiatry to label and deal with people on behalf of society at large' (Brown. 1990).

So, what criteria are we using when we diagnose someone as suffering from a 'mental illness'? I will use 'schizophrenia' as an example, since it has been described as 'the prototypical psychiatric disease' (Boyle, 2002a); any critiques that apply to this condition will have even more force in relation to others whose status as illnesses is less widely accepted.

DSM IV lists some of the diagnostic criteria for 'schizophrenia' as follows:
- flat or grossly inappropriate affect
- digressive, vague, over-elaborate, or circumstantial speech
- unusual perceptual experiences
- marked lack of initiative, interests or energy
- markedly peculiar behaviour (eg. collecting garbage, talking to self in public, hoarding food)
- marked impairment in personal hygiene and grooming

- odd beliefs or magical thinking, influencing behaviour and *inconsistent with cultural norms* [my italics]

This list may well describe someone whom we would instinctively recognise as having serious problems, which is partly where it gets its credibility from; clearly, *something* is wrong. But the key question is whether that 'something' is best described within a biomedical model as an *illness*, that is, only or primarily in terms of biological pathology.

There are two main requirements for the diagnosis of an illness. The first is the identification of particular clusters of *symptoms*, which are the complaints that people go along to their doctor with, such as 'I feel nauseous/tired/in pain'. Since these are largely subjective, diagnosis can only be confirmed by a consistent association with *signs* such as measures of blood sugar, white blood cell counts, abnormalities that show up on x-rays and so on, which are objectively verifiable by others (Boyle, 1999). Notoriously, no such signs are available for psychiatric diagnosis (with a few exceptions such as dementia). You cannot use an x-ray or blood test to tell if someone really is suffering from a biological illness which we can call 'schizophrenia'; thus, in medical terms, we are not justified in asserting that such a condition either exists or has been identified.

However, the problem goes deeper than this. What we are offered instead, in DSM and the International Classification of Diseases (ICD), is an exhaustive list of 'symptoms' which, as a moment's thought will reveal, are actually nothing of the kind. DSM criteria such as those listed above are not complaints about bodily functioning. They are examples of *beliefs, experiences and behaviour,* for which there can be no absolute and agreed standards of 'normality'. While it is relatively simple, in principle, to work out how the body ought and ought not to function, it is an entirely different matter to decide how people ought and ought not to think, feel and behave. How flat or inappropriate does your affect have to be? How digressive, vague and over-elaborate is too digressive, vague and over-elaborate? Exactly how unusual are your perceptual experiences? How much energy or initiative should you have? How much garbage have you collected? How long is it since you last had a bath? These are social not medical judgements, as indeed is openly admitted at several points in DSM ('... inconsistent with cultural norms'). We may have identified troubled or troubling individuals; we have certainly not identified medical illnesses. The criteria for making these decisions are essentially subjective, based on personal and social norms, and thus, in their own terms, unscientific.

A number of consequences follow from having a system of social judgements dressed up as medical ones, which constitutes a kind of parody of the diagnostic process in other branches of medicine. Perhaps most damaging to psychiatry is the consistent failure to demonstrate that psychiatric classification is either reliable or valid, which again is crucial to claims of scientific respectability.

Readers are referred to other sources for a more detailed discussion (Kutchins & Kirk, 1999; Boyle, 2002b); but, in brief, reliability refers to the likelihood that different clinicians will come up with the same diagnosis when presented with the same patient. If psychiatric judgements are essentially subjective, agreement is bound to be low, as has been found (Kirk & Kutchins, 1994). Successive editions of DSM and ICD can be understood as attempts to increase reliability by adding yet more and more detailed criteria; however, if the underlying problem of the subjective nature of the judgements involved is not resolved, then this manoeuvre is doomed to failure.

Even if reliability were to be established, this is not the same as demonstrating that the term that clinicians have agreed upon is meaningful, or valid, actually representing something in the real world. In the 17th century there was widespread agreement on how to identify witches; this does not mean that witches (or 'schizophrenics') actually exist anywhere except in our own heads.

Finally, the lack of reliability or validity of the concept of 'schizophrenia', as well as every other psychiatric diagnosis, undermines any and all research that takes such terms as given. One cannot hope to produce anything but confusing and contradictory results if the validity of basic terms has not been established. This is 'a massive flaw in every single study undertaken' (Hill, 1993).

Space does not allow for a more detailed discussion of the consequences of psychiatric diagnosis such as stigma, medicalising of social and relationship problems, overuse of physical interventions and so on, which I have documented elsewhere (Johnstone, 2000). Indeed, if Brown is right that 'the critique of psychiatry *is* the critique of diagnosis', and if the above critique is accepted, then I have fulfilled my aim of demonstrating the illegitimacy of psychiatry's status as a branch of medical science, with all the consequences that follow from that. However, I would like to extend and elaborate on the argument by looking at the two other principal arguments for understanding distress within a biomedical framework, that is, by examining claims about the biochemical and genetic origins of mental distress.

Biochemical causation

As we have seen, it is commonly stated as a fact that conditions such as 'schizophrenia' or 'depression' are caused by 'biochemical imbalances'. As a further twist it is claimed that medication and ECT work by rectifying these 'imbalances'. For example, an advice columnist who describes herself rather misleadingly as a 'holistic doctor' writes, in a popular women's magazine: 'Depression is an unpleasant condition that…is caused by an imbalance of certain chemicals in the brain … Your GP may recommend antidepressants, which work by correcting the chemical imbalance' (Brewer, 1999).

Such statements refer to the actions of neurotransmitters, chemicals in the brain and nerve cells that carry messages between cells by travelling across the gap, or synapse, between them. It is believed that mood is regulated by neurotransmitters (among their many other functions), although this theory is, in itself, speculative. In fact, we know very little about the extraordinarily complex ways in which the brain and its 200-plus transmitters work, and there is no good reason why dopamine and serotonin have become the neurotransmitters of choice in biomedical explanations of mental distress; any of the others, about which we know even less, might be equally suitable candidates.

Confident statements about biochemical causation fail to take account of some rather serious practical problems. Among these are:

1   There is currently no way of directly studying or measuring neurotransmitter levels in the live human brain.

2   Even indirect measurements, via metabolites in the blood or urine, have failed to find evidence of altered neurotransmitter levels in people with a psychiatric diagnosis (Colbert, 2001a).

3   To talk about the action of serotonin (or any other neurotransmitter) in this way is an enormous over-simplification. It has been estimated that there are 100 billion neurones in the brain, each of which may be communicating by chemical transmission with tens of thousands of others, making some 100 trillion synapses in total (Rose 2005). Moreover, different connections have different effects and purposes, and there may be many types of receptor for each neurotransmitter (more than a dozen for serotonin, for example). We are a very long way from being able to make precise and definite statements about how any of these transmitters work.

4   The information that we do have about neurotransmitter action suggests that the phrase 'biochemical imbalance' is fairly meaningless anyway. Neurotransmitters are in a constant state of flux and change as the body seeks to regulate its functions (a process

known as homeostasis); they do not get knocked out of balance at some arbitrary level like a bicycle getting stuck in third gear. A perfect state of balance would be death.

There are also some serious logical difficulties with statements about biochemical imbalances. The basic confusion is between *correlation* and *causation*, an important distinction which is fundamental to scientific reasoning. Even were it to be established that, say, a low mood is consistently accompanied by, or correlated with, lower levels of serotonin, this would not prove that the biological state led to, or caused, the mental one. The causal link might work the other way around; perhaps the mental state of depression leads to the change in biochemistry, rather as fear results in the production of adrenaline.

Another possibility is that some third factor common to both the mental and the physical state is playing a causal role. The obvious third factor is medication, and any methodologically sound study needs to take its effects into account. Thus, in investigating differences between 'schizophrenics' and 'normals', your first group needs to be drug-free, or else you will not be able to tell whether differences are related to the condition or to the treatment. An astonishing number of studies are invalidated by this absolutely basic flaw, including those that have found a greater number of dopamine receptors in the brains of those with a diagnosis of 'schizophrenia' (Colbert, 2001a).

While psychiatry's simplistic claims about biochemical causal mechanisms are unfounded, it would be a mistake to fall into the opposite trap of assuming that there is no link between our bodies and our minds. Indeed, it is increasingly recognised that emotional factors such as attachment styles and trauma have profound effects on the way the brain develops, which in its turn influences an individual's responses and reactions – but this is a highly sophisticated interaction, not a simple one-way link from brain to behaviour (Balbernie, 2001; Schore, 2001). Research shows that the infant brain only develops to its full potential in response to the intimate relationship with its caregiver, which leads directly to the production of new synapses and the creation of new neural pathways. Conversely, detrimental early emotional experiences can cause neurobiological damage that leaves a lifelong biologically based impairment in regulating impulse and emotion. 'Maltreatment can physically alter the wiring and chemistry of the brain' (Balbernie, 2001: 245), although the right environment (which might include psychotherapy and other kinds of re-learning) can repair some of this damage (Carlowe, 2002). As our knowledge increases, we need to find a way of including such biological variables into our understandings, without falling back into reductionist and determinist fallacies.

Biochemical arguments and the use of medication

Ironically, there is one way in which the idea of a 'biochemical imbalance' does make some sense, and that is in explaining the effects of psychiatric drugs. We may know very little about biochemical causal mechanisms in mood and behaviour, but we do know something about the effects of introducing drugs into the body. When neuroleptics block the receptors whose job it is to pick up the chemical messages, then according to the well-established principle of homeostasis, the body will try and compensate for this change by making more receptors and/or increasing the sensitivity of the existing ones. Similarly, when antidepressants prevent the body from sweeping up excess serotonin in the synapse, then some serotonin receptor cells will die off because fewer are needed to detect its presence. Now we really do have something that could be described as a 'chemical imbalance', which shows itself very unpleasantly through the side-effects of psychiatric drugs, and also through withdrawal effects, as the body struggles to adjust to the lack of a substance which it had made adaptations to cope with. 'Putting any new chemical into the body is the real equivalent of a spanner in the works, and is likely to have multiple effects – both wanted and unwanted' (Rose, 2005: 230).

These embarrassing facts about the way psychiatric drugs 'work' have been presented in a rather different way by psychiatrists, who commonly argue that because drugs reduce levels of dopamine (or increase levels of serotonin), then excess dopamine/insufficient serotonin is a cause of 'schizophrenia'/depression. It is the known effect of drugs on dopamine and serotonin that has led to the popularity of these neurotransmitters in theories of biochemical causation. However, this kind of argument from effects to causes is illogical and unscientific. It is rather like saying that because aspirin relives headaches, headaches must be caused by a lack of aspirin in the brain.

In a variation on this theme, lay people sometimes say, 'If it isn't an illness, how come the drugs seem to help?' This too is confusing cause with effect. Of course the drugs have an impact, but they have an impact on anyone, whether psychiatrically diagnosed or not (as the occasional accounts of non-diagnosed people who have taken psychiatric drugs tell us, for example, Jones-Edwards, 1993). This doesn't tell us anything about the causes of distress. The effects of the drugs are non-specific; along with reducing 'symptoms' for some people, they lessen your ability to think and feel in all areas of your life. While some may experience this as helpful, it does not address the underlying problem any more than taking a tranquilliser to cope with the anguish of bereavement. Moreover, there are very serious consequences to this kind of 'help', including long-term biological changes leading to tardive dyskinesia and many other types of damage (Breggin, 1993).

Summary

In summary, to state that 'mental illness is caused by biochemical imbalances' is, to put it at its best, completely without supporting evidence. 'There is no known lowering of serotonin in depression ... No one for whom Prozac has been prescribed has ever had their serotonin levels checked to see if the really are suffering from what the drug supposedly corrects' (Healy 1998). If you go along to your GP complaining of a low mood, he/she does not check your serotonin levels, confirm the diagnosis, and ask you to return in three weeks for another test to see if medication has restored them to the correct level; it just doesn't work like that. Moreover, the information that we do possess suggests that such a theory is ludicrously simplistic. The brain 'beggars in complexity even the most intricately engraved silicon ship' (Rose, 2005: 146); and 'There is not and cannot be any straightforward one for one relationship between the complexities of our mental experiences and the simplicity of a single biochemical measure' (Rose, 2005: 237).

Tacit acknowledgement of these embarrassing holes in the evidence can sometimes be detected in weaker forms of the theory, expressed as 'Neurotransmitters are *thought to be* involved with major depression' (NAMI information leaflet, 2003) or 'Schizophrenia is ... *probably* due to physical and biochemical abnormalities in the brain' (Orion Pharma, 1995) [my italics]. However, such statements are virtually meaningless in scientific terms. Neurotransmitters are involved in everything we think, feel or do. One could argue, with equal validity, that they are 'thought to be involved' in watching television, chatting to the neighbours and brushing your teeth. Proper scientific hypotheses have to be open to proof or disproof, whereas 'the belief that the "true" biochemistry of schizophrenia is complex and will not be quickly discovered ... is untestable: To say that an unknown number of biochemical substances may interact in an unknown way to produce schizophrenia is a tortuous way of admitting that we have no clue as to what the hell is going on' (Skrabanek, 1984). In fact, it becomes an article of faith, not a valid scientific proposition at all.

Genetic causation

It is almost universally accepted that there is an important genetic contribution to 'schizophrenia', and probably to other serious psychiatric conditions as well, although it is acknowledged that environmental factors play a part as well. Sometimes genetic and biochemical theories are linked; for example, it is said that the faulty gene(s) may lead to irregularities in dopamine production. Breakthroughs in discovering the relevant genes are regularly announced in the newspapers, although the inevitable retractions get a more limited press: 'Scientists seeking genetic link to mental illness "draw blank"' (*The Independent*, 1998). 'We are sort of back to square one' (Dr. Kenneth Kidd, quoted in Goode, 2000).

The search for a single gene for 'schizophrenia' or other conditions has been replaced by a recognition that the situation is bound to be more complex than this, and researchers now talk about multiple contributing genes. However, even this hypothesis faces as many practical and logical hurdles as the claims about biochemistry. Once again, I shall use 'schizophrenia', the most researched condition and the one about which the strongest claims have been made, as an example.

As with brain biochemistry, our knowledge of genetics is still very limited. Although scientists have recently completed the enormous task of decoding the human genome, or in other words, making a list of the sequences of all the pieces of DNA that make us the living creatures that we are, some experts have suggested that we are at least a century away from actually understanding what all of this means and how it works. We have painstakingly copied out a massive book whose language is still largely incomprehensible to us. What we do know suggests that the processes involved are extremely complex; each gene may make several proteins, and each protein may perform more than one job. Conversely, a whole number of genes may interact to produce a single physical characteristic. Intriguingly, there may also be a greater role for the environment than had been suspected, since scientists have found that we possess far fewer genes than originally assumed. This 'dramatically undermines claims that human beings are prisoners of their genes' (McKie, 2001).

So far, scientists have only been able to identify specific genes for a very small number of conditions such as cystic fibrosis and Huntingdon's chorea, but these relatively simple forms of transmission, in which it does make sense to talk about a gene or genes for a certain condition, are certainly untypical.

Practical problems with backing up claims about genetic transmission in 'schizophrenia' include the following:

1   No gene or set of genes has been identified for any mental illness.
2   Announcements about 'breakthroughs' refer not to the supposed discovery of genes themselves, but to markers, indicators that certain genes may (or may not) be found nearby. Identifying a marker is a long way from finding the possible defective gene that may be associated with it – it took ten years to move from marker to gene in the case of Huntingdon's chorea. No markers for any mental illness have ever been found, and even if they had been, this would not necessarily imply the existence of a gene for the condition.
3   In the absence of such findings, statements about genetic contributions to 'schizophrenia' rely on data from family, twin and adoptive studies, all of which seem to show that it 'runs in families'. However, this could obviously be a result of environmental factors (family relationships, social stresses etc) instead of genetics. In practice, it is almost impossible to untangle the nature/nurture contribution, and the key studies that claim to do so are riddled with basic methodological problems, which there is no space to discuss in detail here (but see Colbert, 2001b; Joseph, 2004; Marshall, 1990; Boyle, 2002b; Rose, Lewontin & Kamin, 1990). In general, the more rigorous the study, the smaller the genetic contribution that emerges. One reviewer has noted: 'That the reported studies are riddled with methodological, statistical and interpretational errors has repeatedly been demonstrated' (Sarbin, 1991). Another writes: 'This is not science. This is simply the *mathematical manipulation of meaningless* data' (Colbert, 2001b) [italics in original].
4   The data from this research do not conform to any known pattern of inheritance. One often cited study appeared to show that half-siblings were more likely to develop the condition than full ones (Breggin, 1993: 119). Nor do inheritance rates seem to have been reduced by the policy of incarcerating people in asylums throughout their reproductive years, or indeed by the mass extermination of psychiatric patients in Germany during the Second World War.
5   Finally, and most importantly, claims about genetics all founder on the fact that, as already discussed, *there is no known biological abnormality in schizophrenia or any other psychiatric condition.* It is clear what is, or could be, inherited in physical diseases such as cystic fibrosis. In the case of psychiatric conditions we are, as we saw when we discussed diagnosis, talking not about physical malfunctioning but about *beliefs, experiences and behaviour.* It is not at all obvious how these could be passed on in the genes, even in principle.

Genetic arguments, like biochemical ones, have their fair share of logical difficulties too. The correlation/causation problem applies here as well; even had we got as far as identifying genes that were consistently associated with psychiatric conditions, we would still not know whether the first caused the second, or whether this was just a chance association. Researchers would have to be able to point to a biological change associated with the mental 'illness' and show how the gene(s) led to this specific change. As we know, no such biological change has been found.

However, as noted above, the most serious difficulty with genetic theories is the assumption that beliefs, experiences and behaviour can somehow be determined by genes. The link from genes to behaviour is almost infinitely long and complex, and includes all the developmental, environmental, social and cultural influences that a human being is exposed to, not to mention their own capacity to make sense of all these and exercise free will in deciding for themselves how to react. Also, descriptions of problematic behaviour are socially defined; it makes no sense to talk in the abstract of 'delusions' or 'withdrawal' as pathological entities without looking at the context in which they are occurring. Some unusual beliefs are widely shared and hence not considered abnormal, while withdrawing from others, collecting garbage, hoarding food and so on are all understandable in certain circumstances. Professor Steven Rose has discussed the flaws in the current fashion for what he calls 'neurogenetic determinism', the idea that our genes determine our behaviour. A committed scientist himself, he concludes that this is simply a case of faulty reasoning and bad science (Rose, 1998). In other words, as a speaker from the Genetic Forum in London puts it, 'The idea that human behaviour can be explained at a molecular level is patently rubbish' (Jenkins, quoted in Boley, 1995).

We can take this argument further. Let us suppose, leaving aside for the moment all the problems with diagnosis, that more methodologically sound family and adoption studies do consistently suggest a small but significant hereditary factor in 'schizophrenia'. Even this would not necessarily imply an illness with a primarily genetic component, because what is inherited might be something less specific, such as a general sensitivity to environmental stresses. This characteristic might be widely distributed in the general population and only disadvantageous in certain circumstances.

Interestingly, this is precisely the conclusion that was tentatively put forward by the Finnish authors of a recent and more sophisticated adoption study. In comparing adopted children whose mothers had a diagnosis of 'schizophrenia' with another group of adoptees without such a history, they found that the genetic background only resulted in breakdown when combined with disturbed family environments. All children, in either group, did well in 'healthy' families. They concluded, firstly, that environmental not genetic factors may be the crucial factor in leading to, or protecting from, serious breakdown; and secondly, that what is inherited may be a non-specific sensitivity. 'If this turns out to be the case, the diagnosis of schizophrenia as a specific disease entity may also need revision' (Lehtonen, 1994).

Summary

In summary, I have argued that there is no scientific evidence, and indeed could not in principle be any evidence, for the proposition that 'there is a gene/are genes for mental illness'. Nor does the basic assumption behind such arguments, that genes can in some way be partialled out from the environment, make sense. Genes can only be expressed via the environment – and this is true at all levels, from the cellular metabolic system that surrounds an individual piece of DNA right up to the social and cultural world that the person inhabits. We saw this in the earlier discussion about brain development. Even identical twins will show differences according to their position in the womb. 'The very concept of unpicking genes and environment misspeaks the nature of developmental processes. The developing foetus, and the unique human being which it is to become, is always both 100 per cent a product of its DNA and 100 per cent a product of the environment of that DNA – and that includes not just the cellular and maternal environment but the social environment in which the pregnant mother is located ... The "environment" impinges from the moment of conception' (Rose, 2005: 61, 59).

Vulnerability-stress models of mental distress

As with biochemical theories, there are strong and weak versions of the orthodox position on the genetics of 'mental illness'. A popular current model claims that genes play a predisposing role, with environmental factors triggering the actual appearance of the condition. Variations on this are known as the 'vulnerability-stress' or the 'stress-diathesis' or the 'biopsychosocial' model (Zubin & Spring, 1977) and are subscribed to by most researchers and clinicians today. These will be discussed below.

It is important to be clear what might be implied by these terms. In one sense, such hybrid models are obviously true, hence their plausibility. Genes, like neurotransmitters, are involved in some way and at some level in everything we think, feel or do; we could not think without having inherited a brain to think with, nor could we act without having inherited bodies to carry out our actions. Similarly, it is only commonsense to agree that almost every condition that humans can experience is an end result of biological, psychological and social factors. You could equally well argue that such a model 'explains' why someone enjoys music, rides a bicycle, and drinks tea. However, as with the equivalent biochemical theories, this actually tells us nothing at all.

What needs to be established by supporters of this watered-down version of the biomedical model is that genes or biology make a *significant primary causal contribution,* such that it makes sense to describe mental distress as an 'illness'. As we have seen, evidence for the 'vulnerability' or the 'bio' bit of the model, that is, the bit that involves the identification of a biological malfunction or associated genes, is entirely lacking. As far as we know, the models are only true in the very weak sense outlined above, but to assert this is, in scientific terms, virtually meaningless.

Meaningless; but not purposeless – under the guise of open-mindedness and commonsense, psychiatrists have been able to perpetuate the assumption that biological processes are the most important explanatory factors, in the face of increasing evidence for environmental ones. Moreover, in vulnerability-stress models the environmental factors are reduced to a 'triggering' role which entirely deprives them of their personal meaning and significance. Why does a bereavement, or job loss, or abuse in childhood lead to breakdown in one person and not another? Such questions cannot even be asked, let alone answered, within a model that reduces everything apart from biology to a mere 'trigger', to be bracketed off while medication deals with the 'real' underlying problem. This weak version of positivist psychiatry leaves the patient in essentially the same position as the 'strong' biomedical one, 'for it too denies that the patient's response to his or her surroundings is intelligible and *valid*' (Ingleby, 1980b: 45) [italics in the original].

An interesting illustration of this comes from the well-known field of research into expressed emotion (EE) in 'schizophrenia', which is firmly situated within a vulnerability-stress model of psychosis. It has been well established that high levels of EE in a family (hostility, critical comments, and over-involvement) lead to an increased risk of relapse in the identified patient. Treatment packages have been developed which aim to reduce the levels of EE in a family and hence of relapse, by problem solving, developing better communication skills, spending time apart and so on (Fadden, 1998). Significantly, the one thing that professionals are strongly discouraged from doing is looking too deeply at the *meaning* of all this EE. ('We do *not* view the family as in need of treatment. Hence we avoid calling our interventions "family therapy". Our aim is to help the family to cope better with the sick member who is suffering from a defined disease' (Kuipers, Leff & Lam, 1992)). However, research by Harrop and Trower (2003) suggests that the interactions that take place under the heading of EE are far from a simple accumulation of unpleasant remarks. In-depth interviews with the identified patients revealed that it is the *personal meaning* of the interactions that makes them so upsetting; more specifically, when others' comments are experienced as a threat to one's identity and preferred view of oneself. This dimension is entirely lost in a strict vulnerability-stress model which simply sees criticism as the trigger for an underlying disease process.

Discussion

> I just *know* that the biological approach to psychological distress is bollocks
>
> Smail, 1996: 16

'Just *knowing*' is, of course, not enough in scientific terms, no matter how sympathetic we may be to the sentiment expressed. However, we have now assembled enough arguments to conclude that supporters of a biomedical model of distress are themselves on no firmer ground. Anyone approaching the evidence, or lack of it, from an impartial angle would surely conclude that it actually constitutes strong support for a non-medical understanding of distress as arising from environmental factors. But no matter what the research turns up, the theory survives because supporters just *know* it is true. This is despite the admission in some very respectable circles that things are not as clear-cut as other sources lead us to believe:

> In some quarters schizophrenia has gained the reputation of a graveyard of research. Few findings stand the test of time, most of the pieces of this particular jigsaw seem to be missing, and it is not easy to make sense of those that are available. Even 'hard' scientific findings fail to be replicated.
>
> Mortimer, 1992

> The precise causes of most mental disorders are not known...No single gene has been found to be responsible for any specific mental disorder ... There is no definitive lesion, laboratory test or abnormality in brain tissue that can identify mental illness.
>
> US Department of Health and Human Services, 1999

The intriguing question is how and why such theories survive. To the non-specialist, the scientific language carries an aura of respectability that presumably once accrued to religious explanations ('He is possessed by evil spirits'), although the current belief that people are, in effect, 'possessed by schizophrenia' is no better founded, as will become apparent to anyone brave enough to ask for details. As a service user said to me, 'A relative asked, well if it's a biochemical imbalance, which is the chemical imbalanced in Joan? And Dr Smith looked at her absolutely speechless and said, on well, it doesn't work like that ... I don't honestly believe that they know what they're doing, I honestly don't.'

It is more puzzling when these explanations are put forward by people whose professional training must tell them that they are talking nonsense. As Mary Boyle puts it, 'How is the presentation of "schizophrenia as a brain disease" managed in such a way that the absence of direct evidence will not be noticed or seem important?' (Boyle, 2002b: 9). She gives examples of a number of strategies that are used either consciously or unconsciously. These include the simple assertion that this is the case (eg. the quotes at the start of the chapter); omitting to mention critiques; listing apparently meaningful associations between biological factors and specific diagnoses (although these are at best correlational and not causal); minimising the role of psychosocial factors, or else attributing them to the 'mental illness' itself; using medical analogies such as diabetes; and so on.

This gives us some clues as to *how* biomedical theories survive. A discussion about *why* they do so is beyond the scope of this chapter (see following chapter by Terry Lynch), and would have to include the position of those who may be relieved to find a way of escaping from guilt, shame and painful personal exploration; the professional interests of those whose career and status are predicated on these theories; and the enormously powerful business interests of the pharmaceutical companies (Johnstone, 2000). Several of the authors cited earlier are clear that a full answer must also include the wider *political* usefulness of such theories. 'The motivations for such reductive explanations derive ... from the urgent pressure to find explanations for the scale of social and personal distress in advanced industrial societies ... Reductionist ideology serves to relocate social problems to the individual, thus "blaming the victim"' (Rose, 1998: 296). 'Biological psychiatry has always had to perform social functions that are supportive of established authority, especially in times of marked social inequality or entrenchment ... Human choices and values are negated, and the sociocultural status quo remains intact' (Pam, 1995: 3). 'The inappropriateness of the positivist paradigm, in rational terms, is precisely what makes it so appropriate to the task of preserving existing institutions from the threat of change ... Radical politics, and the undermining of psychiatry, are thus inseparable from each other' (Ingleby, 1980b: 45).

But to return to the start of the argument, the problem facing the biomedical model of mental distress runs deeper than mere lack of evidence, crucial though this is, or bad science, endemic though that also is in psychiatric research and reasoning. The fundamental problem is the inappropriateness of positivist, reductionist and deterministic models to explain human experience. We urgently need new and radically different paradigms for understanding and responding to mental distress, or, as I would prefer to call it, human suffering; models that incorporate a holistic understanding about what it is to be human, and a full acknowledgement that our distress has both meaning and purpose.

Moral philosophers have long contended that 'morality depends ... on our ability to treat one another always as persons ... Moral relations are dependent on the absolute value of a human being, as a free human spirit' (Macmurray, 1935). As psychologists have also noted, seeing people as objects is the necessary first step that allows us to treat them in ethically unacceptable ways (Williams, 1992). The biomedical model of mental distress sets the scene for this by depriving people of their personhood, agency and personal meanings. We can, I believe, see ample evidence of the inevitable consequences of this in biomedical psychiatry: consistent protests from service users that they are unheard and treated without dignity or respect; decades of interventions (emetics, purgatives, rotating chairs, straitjackets, incarceration, solitary confinement, lobotomy, insulin coma, unmodified ECT) that are better described as torture than treatment; and the appalling neurological damage inflicted on millions of the world's most vulnerable people by the indiscriminate use of neuroleptics and other drugs. That is why questions about how we respond to human suffering are not simply ones of science or evidence, though that may be a part of it. They are ultimately moral, ethical and political issues on which we all need to take a stand.

Acknowledgement

Many thanks to Donnard White and Anneke Westra for their detailed comments on this chapter.

6

Understanding Psychiatry's Resistance to Change

Terry Lynch

I have been a fully registered GP, based in Limerick, Ireland, for over twenty years. I re-trained as a psychotherapist, in an attempt to fill the gaping holes in my medical training regarding how to deal with emotional and mental distress. My book, *Beyond Prozac: Healing mental suffering without drugs* (Lynch, 2001) was published in Ireland in April 2001. Six thousand copies have been sold in Ireland up to June 2003, a country whose population matches that of Manchester. *Beyond Prozac* was short-listed for the MIND Book of the Year award in 2002, and a second edition was published in the United Kingdom by PCCS books in 2004. Dorothy Rowe wrote the foreword.

For generations, the medical profession has been given prime responsibility for mental health care. Governments throughout the world see no need to assess independently the validity of the claims and the practices of psychiatry. This is, I believe, a serious error on the part of governments worldwide. Are psychiatrists and GPs truly the independent thinking, objective scientists they portray themselves to be? Lets look for a moment at what doctors say, and compare that to what they do.

The predominant belief within the medical profession regarding mental health problems such as depression, bipolar disorder and schizophrenia, is that these so-called 'mental illnesses' are physical, biological problems requiring physical, biological treatments. Doctors frequently compare these so-called 'mental illnesses' to biochemical conditions such as diabetes. The experience of one client of mine illustrates this common practice. This man, in his early thirties, attended his GP six months ago. My client had been attending that practice intermittently for two years, during which time his distress had been interpreted as depression, and he had been put on antidepressant medication. On this occasion, this man attended the GP to have his headaches checked out. He did not want his GP to get involved in his distress. He was coming to me about that. We had built up a trusting relationship, and we were making progress together.

The GP's reaction is typical of how the medical profession sees and deals with emotional distress. My client told the GP that he was there to have an organic cause for his headaches ruled out, and no more. On hearing that my client was on only a relatively moderate dose of an older type antidepressant, the GP launched into a lecture; 'Depression is caused by a biochemical abnormality. You're only fooling yourself if you think you can talk your way out of depression. Eventually you will see sense and come around to our way of thinking.'

This person came to me the following day, distressed and angry at the manner in which he had been treated by the GP. As we spoke, I asked him if he would like me to ring the GP in his presence to clarify matters. He asked me to do so, and the GP confirmed on the phone to me that he had said these exact words to this man. When I asked the GP what tests he had carried out to confirm this person's biochemical abnormality, the GP told me that I was being petty. Incidentally, this man was fully off medication within two months of the GP insisting he needed a much higher dose of medication. He has now made an excellent recovery from what was an enormously painful degree of emotional distress which was simplistically labelled as 'depression' by his GP.

Neither GPs nor psychiatrists ever confirm any psychiatric diagnosis with laboratory tests. The GP referred to above did not carry out any tests to confirm his confident assertion that this man had a biochemical brain abnormality. Why? Because no such tests exist. If such tests did exist, they would immediately become widely publicised and widely available. Those who support the biomedical approach would ensure that they became widely available. Such tests would enormously vindicate the biomedical approach.

Compare this to what doctors do regarding known biochemical conditions such as diabetes. Biochemical tests are an essential part of the diagnosis and ongoing management of diabetes, and of all known biochemical conditions such as hypothyroidism, pernicious anaemia. No doctor would dream of diagnosing diabetes without the appropriate chemical tests. Yet all doctors who state that depression, bipolar disorder and schizophrenia are caused by a biochemical abnormality, do so without any biochemical tests to verify such claims. It is akin to observing the stars through a telescope and claiming to understand the galaxy.

How can it be that there is such a vast discrepancy between what doctors say, and what they do? This leads me directly into two related topics: the limitations of psychiatry, and psychiatry's resistance to change. Doctors are human. While psychiatrists and GPs publicly project an air of science and authority, to understand the vast discrepancy between what doctors say and what they do, one must look at the human side of the medical profession. Doctors are prone to the same insecurities, vulnerabilities, self-interest, biases, limited vision, external influences, defence mechanisms and wishful thinking that can occur in any area of life.

The defensiveness of medicine

This point about the vulnerability of doctors came forcefully home to me five years ago. I had been asked to give a three-hour talk with recently qualified doctors. During this talk, I expressed my concerns about mental health care, and about major inadequacies in the training these young doctors had experienced. At the end of the talk, most of these young doctors were visibly unsettled. Never before had their faith in the medical system been questioned in such a manner. After the meeting, one doctor wryly commented – 'Great! – now we don't know who we are!'

This apparently casual comment helped me to see the role played by the human aspects of doctors in maintaining the status quo within mental health. Psychiatrists, and to a lesser extent GPs, have an enormous investment in the current medical approach to mental health care. In reality, the biology of mental health problems is a belief system. It is a belief system because doctors have such faith in it, even though their patients never, ever have their supposed biochemical imbalance confirmed by biochemical or other tests.

Three characteristics of belief systems include:

a An investment in the continuation of the belief system by those who run and believe in the system.

b A resistance from within the belief system to question the fundamentals of their belief system and to resist such questioning from others.

c A resistance to the exploration and development of other beliefs, beliefs which might challenge or reduce the power and influence of the said belief system.

It can be said of some belief systems that they are not based on logic, but on faith, desire and wish fulfilment. This is true of psychiatry. Belief systems frequently aspire to a future salvation or redemption. With regard to psychiatry, the future salvation is the hoped-for biochemical and biological proof – at some time in the future – of causation for mental health problems. This hoped-for future salvation would lead to the redemption of psychiatry, allowing psychiatry to take its place as the respected medical speciality it so desperately seeks to be.

Who has most to lose if the current drug-dominated and biologically focused psychiatric system were to be expanded to a truly biopsychosocial model of mental health care? Not mental health service users. Service users want help to overcome the distress they are experiencing, to get their lives back on track. They do not have an enormous vested interest in the type of help provided within the services.

It is the service providers who have the most to lose; psychiatrists, GPs, and of course the pharmaceutical industry. Groups or individuals who have a lot to lose tend to resist changes which may diminish their power, influence, status, earning power, sense of identity, regardless of whether such changes might benefit the community generally. Having for decades placed such trust in the biochemical belief system, to acknowledge the palpable limitations of this belief system and the limitations of medication would mean having to acknowledge that psychiatry has for decades demonstrated poor scientific judgement in its approach to mental health problems. Psychiatrists and GPs would have to admit that there really is very little evidence to back up their insistent claims that mental health problems are caused by brain abnormalities. Given the enormous embarrassment this would cause for psychiatrists and GPs, it is not surprising that psychiatry seeks to maintain the status quo, resisting efforts to expand mental health care into a truly holistic, biopsychosocial approach to mental health care problems. It would mean losing face to such a degree that their respectability, their status, would be seriously undermined. So, it is clear that there is a lot at stake for the medical profession.

The path of psychiatric research over the past 100 years confirms this. Filled with a passionate desire to establish psychiatry as a scientific, respectable branch of medicine, for more than 100 years, psychiatrists made a major error of judgement. They first arrived at their conclusion, the outcome which most excited and validated their view of mental health problems, and set up their research to establish that their conclusion was the correct one.

Having decided that 'mental illness' was caused by a physical brain defect, psychiatry has in the main designed research to establish that this is the case. Thus, the cart was put before the horse. Wishful thinking becomes presented as scientific thinking. This approach is highly unscientific. Science demands, of those who purport to be scientists, an open and enquiring mind; rigorous self-examination to ensure that one's own biases are not influencing one's conclusions; and sufficient honesty and humility to acknowledge the possible validity of views contrary to one's own. Science does require us to be open to the possibility that, at some future time, perhaps biochemical and/or genetic imbalances may be identified for mental health problems. Science also requires that we do not come to premature conclusions; unfortunately, that is precisely what the medical profession has done for decades.

A British professor of psychiatry – Professor Thompson of the University of Southampton – wrote in *Medical Dialogue* December 1997 that 'for more than 30 years, the dominant hypothesis of the biological basis for depression has been related to noradrenaline and serotonin'. Commonsense – not to mention science – suggests that to focus so intensely on one hypothesis for over 30 years, to the virtual exclusion of equally valid psychosocial hypotheses, is a questionable practice. This preoccupation with serotonin typifies the blindness which is a regular occurrence within psychiatry. The underlying purpose of this blindness is, I believe, to preserve the biological belief system, to maintain biopsychiatry at the pedestal of the mental health care system. A pitfall for any belief system is that its faith can be blind; blind to its own limitations, and to the value of other possibilities which do not fall within its own belief system. This blindness is perhaps psychiatry's greatest limitation, the ultimate losers being the mental health service users.

The limitations of psychiatry

It is no coincidence that what psychiatrists value – medication, for example – is widely available to patients, while what psychiatry does not value – counselling, self-esteem and self-confidence building, empowerment-building programmes, step-by-step programmes to help people get their lives back on track, for example – are thin on the ground within mainstream mental health services.

There is such widespread faith in medical circles regarding the superiority of antidepressants over other approaches. Yet, there is a great deal of evidence countering this claim. There is considerable evidence that antidepressants may only be marginally more effective than placebo. For example, according to the Cochrane Review, the differences between antidepressants and active placebos are small (Moncrieff et al, 2004). A 1999 study, carried out over a six month period, found a 47 per cent remission rate within the study group who took placebo only just slightly less than the groups who took either mianserin (54 per cent remission rate) or sertraline (61 per cent remission rate) (Malt et al, 1999). A recent US study found that people diagnosed as being depressed actually fared better on a placebo than on either sertraline or St. John's Wort (Hypericum Depression Trial Study Group, 2002).

Studies rarely state clearly whether, at the time of the final evaluation, people are still taking the medication or not. My impression is that they probably are. If so, then the results do not reflect the well-recognised deterioration which can occur when medication is stopped. This frequent deterioration is typically explained by doctors to be due to the recurrence of the 'illness' when treatment is stopped. This view fails to take account of two other possible explanations; withdrawal from the medication, and the fact that the person is no longer taking a mood-altering substance means they are more likely to fully experience their unpleasant feelings. This latter point suggests that the principle action of psychiatric drugs is to numb, to sedate and to reduce anxiety. This numbing, sedating, anxiety-reducing effect has its place in the treatment of mental health care problems, but surely it should not be the all-encompassing panacea it is currently considered to be by the medical profession.

The public naturally presumes that medications have been subjected to comprehensive testing prior to being made available to the public. It appears that this is not always the case. It certainly is not the case regarding antidepressant drugs. Eight years after Prozac was first launched, the US Data Sheet for Prozac stated the following:

> The efficacy of Prozac was established in 5- and 6-week trials with depressed outpatients. The antidepressant action of Prozac in hospitalised depressed patients has not been adequately studied. The effectiveness of Prozac in long-term use, that is for more than 5-6 weeks, has not been systematically evaluated in controlled trials
>
> quoted in Medawar, 1997

Yet, in the eight years up to 1998 since the launch of Prozac, this drug had been widely prescribed for millions of people worldwide for periods of many months and sometimes for years. In 1998, ten years after the launch of Prozac, and approximately eight years after the launch of many other serotonin specific reuptake inhibitor (SSRI) antidepressant drugs, an article in a prestigious medical journal conceded:

> One of the most widely accepted tenets of modern psycho-pharmacology is the value of maintenance [drug] treatment of major depression. And yet this de facto consensus treatment strategy remains largely an article of faith, resting as it does on a tenuous empirical base of a small number of placebo-controlled studies totalling fewer than 600 patients.
>
> Keller et al, 1998

A further example of psychiatry's blindness is psychiatry's reliance on antidepressants as the primary treatment for depression, despite considerable evidence that counselling can be as effective as antidepressants. For example, one study compared generic counselling and antidepressants in the treatment of depression (Chilvers et al, 2001). By generic counselling, the researchers meant 'experienced counsellors, who adopted the counselling approach they believe to be most suitable'. People in the counselling group received six sessions with a counsellor. The researchers found that 'at twelve months follow-up, generic counselling and antidepressants are equally effective in patients with mild to moderate major depression'. The researchers concluded that 'General Practitioners should allow patients to have their preferred treatment'. In this study, it was the experience of the counsellor rather than the type of counselling practised by the counsellor that was the telling factor.

Another study found that two psychological interventions – problem solving and a course of prevention of depression – were effective in reducing the severity and duration of depression and improving mental and social functioning in adults (Dowrick et al, 2000). Many other studies have had similar findings. Professor Ivor Browne, formerly professor of psychiatry at University College, Dublin, has long been a critic of psychiatry's preoccupation with medication. According to him (Browne, 1999), 'there is a well-established body of research demonstrating the effectiveness of counselling and psychotherapy [in the treatment of depression]'.

The fact that counselling can frequently be an effective way to deal with depression raises questions regarding the prevailing biological view of depression. If depression were caused by a biochemical deficiency, how could counselling possibly be an effective treatment for depression? To put this into perspective, let us focus for a moment on diabetes, a biochemical condition to which depression is frequently compared by doctors. For example, according to a highly respected Irish GP, Dr. Muiris Houston (2001), 'Depression, in my view, is no different from diabetes. In one you take insulin and in the other you take Prozac or some other antidepressant. Both substances are simply designed to replace natural chemicals missing from the body.'

To even suggest that counselling could be an effective alternative to insulin would be laughable. No doctor would dream of treating his diabetic patients with counselling alone, nor indeed would his patients expect this. The reason is obvious – there is no way that counselling could have such a significant impact on a known, identified biochemical abnormality such as occurs in diabetes. No doctor would dream of treating diabetic patients with a placebo, since placebo would have little or no impact on the known biochemical abnormality. In contrast, 40-50 per cent of people diagnosed with depression recover on a placebo, a fact which raises serious questions regarding the presumed biological nature of depression.

There are many other significant differences between the medical approaches to diabetes and to depression which doctors seem to gloss over. Repeated blood sugar monitoring is an essential part of the diagnosis, treatment and ongoing monitoring of diabetic patients. In contrast, people on antidepressants never have their serotonin levels measured prior to treatment to assess whether their serotonin levels are normal or abnormal to begin with. They never have their serotonin levels checked while on treatment to see whether their so-called 'abnormal' serotonin levels have returned to normal. It has not been scientifically established what the normal range of serotonin levels actually is; and obviously if we don't know what constitutes 'normal' serotonin levels, our scientific knowledge of 'abnormal' serotonin levels is inevitably seriously deficient.

When treatment with antidepressants is stopped, no attempt is made by the doctor to assess serotonin levels. If antidepressants were working all along by returning one's serotonin levels to normal, what happens to one's serotonin level when antidepressants are stopped? Does it now somehow miraculously remain 'normal' in the absence of treatment? Or does it become 'abnormal' again? The bottom line here is that doctors haven't a clue what happens to our patients' serotonin levels when the drug is stopped because we have no way of measuring our patients' serotonin levels, and we do not know what constitutes 'normal' or 'abnormal' levels. We have no idea whether the patients we treat with antidepressants have a normal, low or raised serotonin level at any stage of the entire process of diagnosis and treatment. And we have absolutely no idea how our patients' serotonin levels are responding to the treatment on an ongoing basis. In 20 years as a medical doctor, I have never, ever heard of a patient anywhere having their serotonin levels checked.

Understanding people's distress

I am not alone in believing that antidepressants are significantly overprescribed. While psychiatrists and GPs portray – to the public and to their patients – the impression that the diagnosis and treatment of depression is based on solid, scientific principles, I have long felt that the prescribing of antidepressants in general is anything but scientific. Recent research papers suggest that I may be correct in this view. One study set out to assess the appropriateness of antidepressant prescribing

(Posternak et al, 2002). Remarkably, the researchers found that as many as 85 per cent of depressed patients treated in an outpatient setting would be excluded from the typical study to determine whether an antidepressant would work. Dr. Mark Zimmerman, the study's lead researcher, commented that 'no one knows for sure whether anti-depressants are effective for most of the patients we treat'.

Further questions regarding the stubborn medical faith in antidepressants were raised in a study carried out in Duke University in America (Babyak et al, 2000). This was a follow-up to a study published the previous year by the same university, which had found that regular exercise relieves major depression as effectively as antidepressant medication (Blumenthal et al, 1999). This follow up study showed that exercise is more effective in the long term that sertraline. The researchers found that, ten months after the initial diagnosis of depression, depressive symptoms returned in only 8 per cent of people treated with exercise only. In contrast, depressive symptoms returned in 38 per cent of those treated with sertraline. An interesting finding of this study was that those treated with a combination of exercise and the antidepressant sertraline had quite a high rate of recurrence of depressive symptoms – 31 per cent, much higher that those treated solely with exercise only.

Antidepressant prescribing has risen drastically over the past decade. In 1993, nine million prescriptions for antidepressants were written in Britain. By 1992, that figure had more than doubled – to over twenty two million. Where does the pressure to prescribe come from? I have repeatedly heard doctors plaintively stating that their patients put them under pressure to prescribe medication for their distress. Having listened to many patients over the past twenty years, my feeling is that while people understandably want their distress eased, many people are reluctant to take medication for their emotional distress. The enthusiasm for antidepressant drugs comes not from the public, but from within the medical profession. The findings of a 1995 UK MORI poll support this view (Priest et al, 1996). Asked what treatment should be offered to people who become depressed, only 16 per cent felt that antidepressants should be prescribed. In contrast, 91 per cent of those surveyed felt that counselling should be available in such circumstances.

Over the years, many people have reported to me that their doctor talked them into taking antidepressants. Psychiatry doggedly insists that antidepressants are definitely not addictive, despite the fact that SSRI antidepressants were never systematically tested for their addictive potential. In contrast to the stubborn medical insistence that antidepressants are definitely not addictive, for years the public has not been convinced. The aforementioned 1995 UK MORI poll found that 78 per cent of the public believed that antidepressants were addictive (Priest et al, 1996). I expect that the people surveyed based their opinions on their own experiences, or on the experiences of people around them. In my opinion, the public is a reliable source, since unlike the medical profession and the pharmaceutical industry, the public has nothing to lose if it were established that antidepressants were addictive. The removal earlier in 2003 from the Seroxat leaflet of the words 'Remember, you cannot become addicted to Seroxat', is a remarkable milestone in the unfolding story of SSRI antidepressants.

Regarding the SSRI antidepressants, I believe we are currently watching the unfolding of a debacle similar to the benzodiazepines, the amphetamines, the barbiturates, all of which were enthusiastically and widely prescribed by a medical profession which did not want to hear about people's enormous difficulty coming off these drugs until belatedly forced to do so by growing anger and concern. It is sobering to recall that in 1967, 23.3 million prescriptions were written for amphetamines in the US alone. Over 12 million Americans took amphetamines on medical advice that year (Breggin, 1994).

Regarding what is called schizophrenia, psychiatry has preoccupied itself with certain aspects, such as hearing voices, so-called delusions, and paranoia, seeing these as meaningless and purposeless evidence of psychosis. Hence, psychiatrists rarely explore or validate these experiences. However, I and others have come to see so-called hallucinations, delusions, paranoia and many other such experiences in quite a different light.

These experiences frequently reveal something important about the person, about their life. I have found that exploring these experiences can be extremely worthwhile. Talking about them is frequently very important to the person, since it not everywhere that they can talk candidly about these experiences. I have also learned that through exploring these experiences, both I and the person experiencing them can come to an understanding of them. This can be quite beneficial for a person who up to now has been told that his/her experiences are meaningless, symptoms of their 'illness'.

I was, therefore, very interested to come across a research study that looked at how willing doctors are to engage with people's so-called 'psychotic' symptoms (McCabe et al, 2002). According to the researchers, 'Doctors have trouble talking to patients about psychotic symptoms'. They analysed 32 consultations between psychiatrists and patients with schizophrenia or schizoaffective disorder at two psychiatric outpatient clinics in London. They found that patients actively attempted to talk about the content of their psychotic symptoms, such as hallucinations and delusions, and the distress associated with these symptoms. However, doctors tend to hesitate and avoid answering the patients' questions, indicating a reluctance to engage with these concerns.

The researchers concluded that proactively addressing patients' distress about their psychotic symptoms may lead to a more satisfactory outcome of the consultation itself and improve engagement of such patients with health care services, the researchers concluded. Extraordinary though it might seem, according to these researchers, 'no research has been published on how doctors engage with these patients with psychotic illness in consultations'. And I won't be holding my breath waiting for mainstream psychiatry to enthusiastically develop this possibility further. Because to do so might threaten the belief system, might produce results which question the fixation with biology and which might suggest that approaches other than medication may have real potential. This is directly against the beliefs of the psychiatric belief system. Such ideas will not be fully developed as long as biopsychiatry dominates mental health care, regardless of any potential benefit for the user of the mental health services.

The value of psychosocial interventions

Research sometimes appears in medical journals which runs contrary to the biopsychiatry belief system. One such study looked at the childhood risk characteristics in children who went on to develop schizophrenia-type problems later in life (Morris & McPherson, 2001). The researchers found a significantly higher incidence of social maladjustment at school; a strong preference for solitary play; self-reported social anxiety at age 13; teacher-reported anxiety at age 15; passivity; social withdrawal; social anxiety; hypersensitiveness to criticism; disciplinary problems; anti-social behaviour; flat affect – that is, seldom laugh or smile, no reaction when praised or encouraged. Very significantly in my opinion, the study found that the more anxious children were, the more likely they were to develop schizophrenia. This is a pattern I have repeatedly observed in people who have been diagnosed as having schizophrenia. These features suggest that a psychosocial hypothesis regarding the causation of schizophrenia is at least as valid as the hypothesised biochemical theory.

However, such a psychosocial hypothesis runs contrary to the psychiatric belief system, the blind faith in biology. Consequently, there is little interest or enthusiasm within mainstream psychiatry for psychosocial hypotheses, or indeed for psychosocial interventions.

Schizophrenia Ireland, a major service user group in Ireland, carried out a survey of service users in 2002. Many interesting findings emerged from that survey. The survey asked respondents about a range of non-medical interventions. The most commonly experienced non-medical interventions included employment training, counselling/psychotherapy, peer group support, and art/music therapy. In each of these areas, an average of over 75 per cent found the intervention to be very helpful, or helpful. Yet the vast majority of psychiatrists insist that counselling or psychotherapy are a waste of time in the treatment of schizophrenia, bipolar disorder, and to a considerable degree, depression. These findings also support my view that the medical profession grossly underestimates the reality that people diagnosed with schizophrenia – and other 'mental illnesses' – are more than a diagnosis; they are real people, with real human needs, hopes and aspirations for their life, including the need to belong, to work, to have hope, to have relationships, to have a meaningful life.

Service users are saying they want these services and find them helpful. Psychiatry, however, is telling service users – and governments – that doctor knows best, that service users' own experiences regarding what helps them cannot be relied upon. Hardly a democratic way to provide services. Psychiatry continues to insist that counselling and psychotherapy and other psychosocial interventions have little role in the management of enduring health problems.

It is not as if drug treatment of schizophrenia is so successful that we can be complacent about the possible value of other treatment options. According to psychiatrist Dr. Trevor Turner (1998) of Homerton Hospital, London. 'Sedation, rather than any genuine anti-psychotic effect, is often the main role of standard anti-psychotics'. In spite of repeated medical claims of advancement in the treatment of schizophrenia, the reality is that recovery rates from schizophrenia have not improved over the past 70 years. World Health Organisation studies suggest that recovery rates from schizophrenia are significantly higher in under-developed countries that in developed countries (Sartorius et al, 1996) In order to maintain the biological belief system, psychiatry needs to remain blind to the possibility that psychosocial approaches have real potential. This situation is hardly in the interests of the users of the mental health services.

Similar limitations apply to psychiatry's treatment of what is called 'bipolar disorder'. Widely presumed by psychiatry to be caused by a biochemical imbalance, patients so diagnosed never have their supposed biochemical problem confirmed by any test. Yet, people diagnosed as having bipolar disorder are routinely informed that their condition is caused by a biochemical imbalance, and that their medication will correct this biochemical imbalance. It is worth noting that MIMS Ireland (2000), a physician's medication manual sent to all doctors in Ireland every month (to which Irish doctors repeatedly refer for prescribing information) states that 'the mechanism of action of lithium is unclear'. Medication is the sole treatment offered to the vast majority of those so diagnosed, and medication certainly does have its place. I repeatedly observe that there is a strong psychosocial element to this condition. The 'highs' are frequently triggered by stress, overwhelm, emotional distress and pain. Yet psychiatry offers these people nothing to help them deal with stress and overwhelm. Many of those attending me, diagnosed with bipolar disorder, tell me the work they are doing with me is far more relevant to their life, their experience and their recovery than the medication-based approach of their psychiatrists.

And so it is that issues which are highly relevant to the person's daily experience, their life and their distress, including the distress of depression, so-called 'schizophrenia' and so-called 'bipolar disorder', remain unnoticed and unresolved. Issues such as fear, terror, anxiety, stress, powerlessness, overwhelm, hurt; insecurity, identity issues, relationship issues, life changes; unresolved losses and grief; self-esteem, self-confidence, unresolved and unexpressed feelings; lack of assertiveness; abuse, abandonment, rejection, humiliation, ridicule, bullying; losing face, loneliness; lack of and fear of love and intimacy, difficult life decisions, self-image issues; fear of failure, fear of success, fear of being invisible to others and for some, fear of being visible; one's own expectations, hopes and dreams and those of others; the gradual accumulation of self-doubt; the angst of having so many choices; the human need to belong, to have purpose; sexuality; issues around sex and relationships; financial issues; the need to find various ways of escaping and withdrawing from the difficulties and challenges of life and indeed from the intensity of one's own feelings; the perceived demands of society that one should pretend, wear a mask, that one should hide one's distress; the anxiety associated with risk-taking in life, especially if one's self-esteem is low; peer pressures; the human need for acceptance, affirmation and reassurance; the human instinctual reaction to protect oneself from overwhelm; the human need for a sense of equilibrium and how this equilibrium gets rocked by various shocks in life; performance anxiety; comparisons between self and others; hopelessness; the human need to trust but fearing being let down if one does trust in people; the challenge of taking responsibility for oneself in a difficult world; counterproductive habits such as procrastination; fear of being with or around people yet not really wanting to be alone either; ostracisation of various types; isolation; life events; the double-edged sword of wanting to get on with one's life but being terrified to do so.

These are some of the real issues which the users of the mental health services have to grapple with on a daily basis, issues which psychiatry has decided are of little relevance to people's mental health problems and their recovery.

Many studies over the years have linked low self-esteem to mental health problems. Low self-esteem is an important factor in depression, bipolar disorder, schizophrenia, eating disorders and other mental health problems. Given how ever-present low self-esteem is for people with mental health problems, commonsense would suggest that raising people's self-esteem might be a promising avenue to research in great detail.

However, this has not happened to any significant degree. Indeed, many doctors who regularly prescribe medication for mental health problems undervalue the significance of self-esteem, do not sufficiently understand self-esteem, and know less about raising it. How can this be, you might wonder. The answer is relatively straightforward; self-esteem is not part of the biological model of mental health, therefore it is not seen as important, and is largely discarded as a possibility worth researching. No profession should have such immense power to channel research and the direction of mental health care towards its own biases without appropriate accountability.

Conclusion

I do believe that medication has a place in easing emotional and mental distress. Sometimes, the degree of distress is so acute, so overwhelming that medication can provide a welcome respite from the seemingly never-ending torrent of pain and distress. But rather than being seen as the central, core part of the treatment as is currently the case, medication should be seen as a interim measure, prescribed in the short- to medium-term, as a method of easing the acuteness of the distress.

At the very least, the public is entitled to accurate information regarding medication and how it works. Since we doctors have no accurate idea what effect any psychiatric medication has on the human brain, in the public interest, doctors must cease misinforming the public. No doctor has ever, ever established a biochemical deficiency in any so-called 'psychiatric patient'. No doctor has ever confirmed with biochemical tests that any psychiatric medication has had a beneficial effect on any 'psychiatric patient's' biochemistry. Therefore, regarding all forms of so-called 'mental illness', doctors must cease telling people that medication will correct their biochemical abnormality. All we can tell with any certainty regarding the effects of psychiatric medication is that they are mood altering drugs. It is time that the medical profession came out and acknowledged this truth publicly.

The medical approach focuses on maintenance, on symptom control rather than on recovery. Far more attention and research should be devoted to those who have recovered, to identify what factors were important in their recovery. This information could be an important part of a comprehensive framework for recovery. Such research would contribute to a far more proactive mental health care policy than currently exists, but it isn't happening to any great extent because it is fundamentally challenging to the biomedical belief system.

Any theory which might potentially enhance our understanding and our approaches to mental health problems should receive appropriate attention. Because of medical tunnel vision in favour of biological theories and against psych/socio/emotional aspects of mental health, such exploration is currently not happening. Even in the top psychiatric hospitals, patients regularly report that there is little for them to do during the day. The day typically revolves around the arrival of the drugs trolley.

Steps need to be taken towards the creation of preventative policies within mental health care, something which is currently virtually non-existent, due in no small part to psychiatry's focus on biology at the expense of psychosocial issues. Thus, the limitations of psychiatry permeate all aspects of mental health. I urge everyone to bring this unacceptable situation to an end. Only then can we create a truly biopsychosocial model of mental health care.

7

The Politics of Psychiatric Drug Treatment

Joanna Moncrieff

The place of drug treatment in psychiatry

It is difficult to overstate the central role that drug treatment plays in modern day psychiatry. Psychiatric hospitals and community mental health team activities revolve around the various rituals of drug treatment. In hospital, where virtually every patient is on at least one psychoactive drug and most are on several, there are the regular drug rounds, as well as more dramatic emergency situations where disturbed people are forcibly drugged. Much discussion and energy among staff is devoted to whether patients are on the right sorts of drugs and to whether or not they are actually taking them. Drugs have become the focus of hospital life in a way that ECT and other physical procedures were in the 1940s and 1950s (Braslow, 1997). In the community, staff are also concerned about whether patients are being compliant with medication. Administering depot medications (by injection) is one of the main tasks of community psychiatric nurses, and again, issues about medication are a central feature of meetings between staff and patients and among staff. Medication changes or non-compliance are usually the first explanation invoked when there are changes in someone's mental state, both in hospital and outside.

There is a strong emphasis on the long-term nature of the need for drug treatment in severe mental disorders. For the major psychiatric disorders, such as schizophrenia and manic depression, it is generally suggested that drug treatment is required indefinitely. Even for other less serious conditions such as depression treated in General Practice, it is recommended that drug treatment is taken for a minimum of four to six months after resolution of symptoms (Royal College of Psychiatrists, 2002).

Academic psychiatry also illustrates the central role that drugs play in psychiatric thought. Psychopharmacology has become a major branch of academic psychiatry, with studies of all aspects of drug treatment accounting for a large proportion of empirical research and publication space. Since the 1950s, a fascination with drugs has also stimulated many of the major aetiological theories about psychiatric illness. The actions of drugs were responsible for the notion that psychiatric illness is due to brain neurotransmitter abnormalities, or 'chemical imbalances'. For example, the dopamine theory of schizophrenia arose directly from the discovery of the actions of some of the early antipsychotic drugs. The monoamine theory of depression was elaborated in conjunction with research into the actions of tricyclic antidepressants. Recent ideas about the role of serotonin in depression and other disorders have been stimulated by the introduction of the selective serotonin re-uptake inhibitor (SSRI) drugs such as fluoxetine. These chemical imbalance models have dominated psychiatric thinking about the nature and aetiology of mental illness since the 1960s and have become widely absorbed by the media and general public.

Almost all drugs in current use have been introduced into psychiatry since the 1950s. Although drug treatment was common before that time, with extensive use of barbiturates and other sedatives and some use of stimulants, it was rarely given much attention. This was because drugs were generally regarded as having only crude effects, usually acting as chemical forms of restraint (Braslow, 1997). However, from the 1950s, drug treatment started to arouse considerable interest. The drugs that were introduced from that time onwards came to be regarded as specific treatments for specific conditions and drug treatment was transformed from something that was given little attention to an activity that was seen as making psychiatry truly scientific (Moncrieff, 1999).

Recent developments

Over the last ten to fifteen years psychiatric drugs have become much more widely prescribed and increasingly familiar to the general public. Drugs such as Prozac and Ritalin have become household names and books about them have become best sellers. This is part of a more general increase in consumption of all types of medicines, indicated by the fact that prescriptions issued increased by 56 per cent between 1988 and 2001 in the United Kingdom. However, increases in the use of psychotropic drugs have contributed disproportionately to this increase, with prescriptions of antidepressants rising by 173 per cent in the ten years between 1991 and 2001 (Department of Health, 2002). The rise in cost has been even more marked since the majority of the increases in prescribing have been for expensive new classes of psychiatric drugs. Thus costs of antidepressants in the UK have risen 700 per cent since 1991. In the United States antidepressants are now the top selling class of prescription drug, with antipsychotics, anti-anxiety agents and stimulants all also ranking highly and/or showing rapidly increasing sales (National Institute of Health Care Management, 2002).

This increase in use of prescribed drugs has been achieved firstly by extending the boundaries of well-established conditions like depression and psychosis. Secondly, lesser known diagnoses such as panic disorder and social phobia have been publicised, and thirdly, drug treatment has started to colonise areas where it was previously thought to be unhelpful such as substance misuse and personality disorder.

How effective are psychiatric drugs?

The question that this chapter will attempt to address, is what accounts for the situation outlined. Is it the intrinsic merits of the drugs themselves, or are there other factors that have promoted the use of drugs for psychiatric disorders? First therefore, let me briefly summarise the evidence for the effectiveness of different classes of psychiatric drugs. There has been considerable debate within psychiatry, and on its fringes, about the benefits of modern day drugs. Several critics have claimed that they are not as effective as claimed, and that the effects they have are achieved in much cruder ways than supposed (Breggin, 1991; Fisher & Greenberg, 1989, 1997). Even mainstream psychiatry acknowledges the limitations of drug treatments, and urges a more cautious and limited approach to their use than is generally witnessed in practice. The recent National Institute of Clinical Excellence (NICE) draft guidelines on depression, for example, recommend that drugs should not be used as a first line treatment for cases of mild depression (National Institute for Clinical Excellence, 2003). It is now widely acknowledged that a large proportion of patients, maybe as many as 50 per cent, fail to respond to antipsychotic drugs and that even for people who do 'respond', gains are usually modest. One of the best known British textbooks of psychiatry even questions the overall benefits of long-term antipsychotic drug treatment (Johnstone et al, 1998).

Antipsychotics

Modern drugs used to treat psychotic disorders were first referred to as tranquillisers and they were felt to be uniquely useful due to their ability to tranquillise or quieten without inducing sleep. They were not at first thought to be specific remedies for the biological abnormalities underlying psychiatric conditions. However, fairly soon after their introduction, they came to be seen as having specific properties although there was no evidence which might have supported this change in thinking (Moncrieff & Cohen, 2005). There is no doubt that 'antipsychotic' drugs (also referred to as neuroleptics) do effectively tranquillise or sedate most acutely disturbed patients, although they are frequently supplemented by other sedative drugs such as the benzodiazepines, which are also very effective for this purpose.

However, the question of whether antipsychotics are effective in the long-term treatment of psychotic conditions, such as schizophrenia, is more complex. There are many studies of long-term treatment that appear to show that people who take antipsychotic drugs have a lower chance of relapse than people who are given placebos as a comparison. In clinical practice there is also a strong belief that patients' conditions worsen after antipsychotic drugs are reduced or stopped. However, there are two substantial problems with concluding from this that drugs have beneficial effects on the long-term course of psychotic disorders. Firstly, relapse is often defined as a small increase in non-specific symptoms, which might include insomnia, agitation and anxiety. These symptoms might occur as part of the well-known withdrawal effects of antipsychotic drugs or might be due to anxiety over changes in drug regimes. Secondly, there is some evidence that the discontinuation of long-term drug treatment might itself induce a relapse (Baldessarini & Viguera, 1995; Viguera et al, 1997). Therefore when long-term drug treatment is stopped, either in ordinary clinical practice, or as part of a placebo controlled trial, events after drug withdrawal cannot be taken as representative of the natural history of the condition. Some authors have speculated that this increased vulnerability to relapse after drug withdrawal might be due to the pharmacological adaptations that are induced in the brain during long-term treatment (Viguera et al, 1997). Since all trials of long-term treatment are discontinuation trials, these considerations effectively undermine the evidence for the benefits of long-term antipsychotic drug treatment.

In addition antipsychotic drugs, both the first generation of drugs so called and the more recent new or 'atypical' antipsychotics, have adverse effects. These are usually designated as side effects, but are actually likely to be intimately related to their mode of sedation or tranquillisation. Older drugs cause syndromes akin to Parkinson's Disease and a mental state usually described as indifference, disengagement or 'zombie-like' feelings (Rogers et al, 1998). Newer antipsychotics cause sedation, obesity and diabetes. Hence the costs of antipsychotic drug treatment are considerable and patients frequent non compliance with them can be seen as a rational response.

Lithium and drugs for manic depressive illness

These drugs are often called 'mood stabilisers' although there is no evidence that they have any such specific properties. Lithium was first proposed for the treatment of mania because it was found to produce calming effects in guinea pigs (Johnson, 1984). Lithium undoubtedly has sedative properties, although its utility as a sedative is limited because of its high toxicity. Therefore antipsychotic drugs appear to be better at treating people with severe mania because higher sedative effects can be achieved without the risk of the life threatening toxic effects that occur with lithium (Prien et al, 1972). Therefore the main indication for lithium is the long-term treatment of manic depression where it is supposed to prevent the recurrences that characterise the condition. However, as with antipsychotics, all the trials of long-term lithium involve lithium withdrawal in at least some patients and the evidence that lithium withdrawal induces relapse is now pretty robust (Maj, 2003). Hence the trials that were thought to demonstrate that lithium prevents relapse cannot do so because patients on placebo were likely to have exceptionally high rates of relapse related to lithium withdrawal. In addition, of two recent placebo controlled trials of lithium prophylaxis, only one showed a difference between lithium and placebo (Bowden et al, 2000, 2003).

Nowadays, various anticonvulsants are marketed for the prophylaxis of manic depression and are often preferred to lithium because of the latter's toxicity. None of these drugs have been shown to be superior to lithium, and in the two comparisons with placebo, one showed no difference (Bowden et al, 2000) and the other showed a small effect on depression only (Bowden et al, 2003).

Many studies of the course and outcome of manic depression have not been able to demonstrate that it has improved since the arrival of lithium and other supposed prophylactic drugs, or that patients on lithium do better than patients who are not on lithium (Moncrieff, 1997). Relapse rates in the drug treated groups in older trials of lithium, and recent trials of lithium and anticonvulsants, are around 40-50 per cent over one to two years which are not better than those that were found in the 1940s (Winokur, 1975).

Antidepressants

There are probably thousands of trials of antidepressants, dating from the late 1950s when the concept of an antidepressant was first proposed. Although these trials are conventionally thought to prove the superiority of antidepressants over placebo, their results are in fact very varied and many of them are negative. Two of the largest and most important early trials of antidepressants, the Medical Research Council sponsored trial in the United Kingdom and the National Institute of Mental Health trial done in the United States, were in fact negative, although this is rarely acknowledged (Moncrieff, 2001).

In addition, there are many ways in which antidepressant trials may give spuriously positive results. Firstly, some negative trials are never published (Melander et al, 2003). Also, within published trials, negative outcomes are often suppressed (Melander et al, 2003). Secondly, although trials are meant to be conducted 'double blind', in practice patients can often distinguish whether they are having the active drug or placebo because of the physiological effects of taking an active drug. Assessors may also be able to tell through reports of side effects. This was likely to be a particular problem in trials of older antidepressants that had profound physiological effects such as sedation. Studies that used 'active placebos' to try and improve blindness found smaller differences between older antidepressants and placebo (Moncrieff et al, 1997). It may be less of a problem with newer antidepressants whose subjective effects seem less pronounced. This may account for why a meta-analysis with new antidepressants which included unpublished trials found very small and clinically irrelevant differences between the drugs and placebo (Kirsch et al, 2002). A meta-analysis of trials of new antidepressants in children also found no effects for most drugs tested (Whittington et al, 2004). Thirdly, long-term studies of antidepressant therapy are likely to be confounded by relapse inducing effects of drug withdrawal as for antipsychotics and lithium (Viguera et al, 1998). Fourthly, depression outcome scales contain many items to do with sleep and agitation that would respond to non-specific pharmacological effects such as sedation.

Antidepressants came from a variety of different pharmacological classes and have a wide array of pharmacological actions. In addition, many drugs that are not conventionally regarded as antidepressants have been shown to have effects on depression comparable to antidepressants or superior to placebo including some benzodiazepines, many antipsychotics, some stimulants such as methylphenidate (Ritalin), some opiates and buspirone (references in Moncrieff, 2001 and Moncrieff & Cohen, 2005). Hence there is no evidence that a specific pharmacological mechanism is effective in depression, and rather it seems that the effects of antidepressants may be accounted for by the expectations raised by being on any active drug and/or non specific pharmacological effects such as sedation or stimulation.

This brief critique of some of the evidence base for psychiatric drugs at least demonstrates that the benefits of these drugs are not clear cut. What I will attempt to do in the rest of this chapter is to examine how the vested interests of three powerful social groups: the pharmaceutical industry, the psychiatric profession and the state, have worked to promote the use of drugs for psychological disorders. It is suggested that the motives of these groups might provide an explanation for why the evidence base for psychiatric drugs has been presented in such a positive light and its deficiencies largely overlooked.

The pharmaceutical industry

The pharmaceutical industry is a hugely successful commercial sector. Drug company profits have long outstripped profits from other top companies, but since the 1980s their superiority has climbed further and further (Public Citizen, 2002). As a commercial enterprise, the industry is bound to endeavour to market its products and attempt to maximise its profits. The question I will examine is how much influence it has exercised in the realm of the treatment of psychological disorders, and to what extent that influence has affected approaches to drug treatment.

The industry was involved in establishing a place for the new drugs that emerged in psychiatry in the 1950s and 1960s (Moncrieff, 1999). For example, Swazey (1974) has described the extensive marketing campaign launched by the company SmithKline French that helped to introduce chlorpromazine (Thorazine) into America in the mid 1950s. The company targeted not only doctors but also state legislators to encourage them to increase the healthcare drug budget. The company's chairman even appeared on national television to promote Thorazine (Swazey, 1974). Healy (1997) has recorded the efforts of several drug companies to market amitripyline in the early 1960s, including the mass distribution by Merck of a pamphlet by an eminent psychiatrist called 'Recognising the depressed patient'.

A recent account of the history of psychiatry describes these activities of the industry approvingly as the 'ultimate force behind the adoption of new drugs such as chlorpromazine' and credits them with transforming psychiatry into a genuine and modern medical specialism (Shorter, 1997).

The last ten years or so has seen intensification and widening of the scope of drug industry activities. Disease awareness campaigns have become an important part of the marketing process. They are often run prior to the launch of a product in order 'establish a need' and 'create a desire' (Pharmaceutical Marketing, 2001). These campaigns include the production of research and editorials highlighting the extent of the problem and the need for treatment, the recruitment of prominent academics and celebrity patients to support the message and appear in the media, and the creation of apparent patient support groups, to give credibility to the campaign (Pharmaceutical Marketing, 2001; Mother Jones, 2002). These campaigns have been most intense in the United States where direct to patient advertising is now legal. They are succeeded by intense promotional campaigns that coincide with the launch of the product. Mother Jones magazine (2002) describes several examples of such campaigns, including SmithKline's campaign to publicise the prevalence and need for drug treatment of Social Anxiety Disorder (SAD). Material disseminated to the media in the campaign claimed that SAD affected 13 per cent of the United States population based on market research conducted by SmithKline. The Diagnostic and Statistical Manual puts the figure at 2 per cent. The company, or its public relations agency, appear to have set up the Social Anxiety Disorder Coalition for the purposes of the campaign and academic psychiatrists working with SmithKline appeared on prime time television and radio shows. A poster with the slogan 'Imagine Being Allergic to People' was splashed across billboards all over the United States. Sales of Paxil, SmithKline's drug that was intended to treat Social Anxiety Disorder, increased rapidly after this campaign, and it became the second best selling antidepressant in the United States. Similar campaigns have been launched by Pfizer to publicise Post Traumatic Stress Disorder in order to market its drug Zoloft and Eli Lily to market Prozac, renamed Sarafem, for Premenstrual Dysphoric Disorder. In all these campaigns, the industry has taken conditions that were previously thought to be uncommon, that were not traditionally associated with drug treatment, and whose legitimacy as medical diagnoses was often disputed. Campaigns to persuade the general public that they might have the disorder, and that drug treatment can help were then constructed.

Other activities focus on expanding the boundaries of better established psychiatric conditions. The Defeat Depression Campaign, conducted in the early 1990s in the United Kingdom, was a campaign organised by the Royal Colleges of Psychiatrists and General Practitioners, but funded to an undeclared extent by Eli Lily (makers of fluoxetine). This aimed to increase rates of detection and treatment of depression in General Practice and claimed that up to 20 per cent of GP attenders were depressed and in need of treatment (Paykel & Priest, 1992). Similar campaigns were run in other European countries and the United States. More recently the drug industry is funding research, publication of literature and numerous conferences on the subjects of early intervention and prevention of psychosis. The popularity of such concepts, fuelled by the attention that the drug industry facilitates, are changing practice with regard to treatment of psychosis. Until recently, good practice would generally demand a period of assessment without drugs, and antipsychotic treatment would only be initiated when it was clearly established that they were necessary. Now, early initiation of drugs is increasingly acceptable, and may soon be demanded.

A development that has increased the power of the pharmaceutical industry to conduct such campaigns and influence demand from patients and practice of doctors, is their increasing control of research. As public funding for research has diminished over the last two decades, an increasing proportion of research into medical drugs, around 70 per cent in total, is now funded by the pharmaceutical industry (Bodenheimer, 2000). Not only is the industry providing funding, but drug trials that used to be conducted largely by academic institutions, are now increasingly conducted by commercial research organisations. These organisations compete with each other and with academic institutions and medical practices for contracts to run trials. Hundreds of such organisations may compete for a contract (Bodenheimer, 2000). Hence commercial considerations are driving the process of research. In addition, the results of these trials are usually presented by the drug company sponsor or on its behalf by commercial medical writing companies. The process of 'ghost writing', whereby prominent academic authors put their names on papers prepared by these agencies, has become widespread in some quarters and is often difficult to recognise. Academic doctors, including psychiatrists have also been found to have numerous other links to drug companies including paid consultancies, ownership of stock and speaker fees, which frequently amount to thousands of pounds or dollars a year (Boyd & Bero, 2000).

There is some empirical evidence about how the involvement of drug companies may distort the design and presentation of psychiatric research, although such evidence is not necessarily easy to pin down. Several authors have demonstrated non-publication of negative studies by industry and selective publication of positive results and neglect of negative outcomes (Melander et al, 2003; Safer, 2002). Safer (2002) also found evidence of distortions of design of studies to benefit the sponsor's drug and of concealment of the source of funding. Compared to research into other medical conditions, psychiatric research may be particularly easily distorted by vested interests because of the lack of objective tests for psychiatric conditions, the subjectivity of outcomes, the likely influence of placebo effects and the natural fluctuations in the course of disorders.

The increasing ubiquity of psychiatric drugs, and the explicit publicity issued by some drug companies conveys a strong message about the origin and nature of psychiatric disorders (see material on the Eli Lilly website at www.lilly.co.uk, for example). The message is a highly reductionist one: that disorders are the consequences of imbalances in brain chemicals that can be rectified, at least partially, by the right sort of drug. The image created is one in which human life can be broken up into discrete elements of individual behaviour or experience, all of which are driven by a specific brain chemical or combination of chemicals. Although the importance of social interventions may be mentioned, it is difficult to reconcile this with the primary message about the biological origin of the problem.

In conclusion, there are grounds to believe that the pharmaceutical industry has a role in shaping the way in which we view the nature of psychiatric disorders, as well as influencing what is regarded as the most appropriate treatment. It is currently helping to stretch the boundaries of what is considered to be a psychiatric disorder, and to expand the justifications for drug treatment. In the process it is reinforcing a narrow reductionist view of psychiatric conditions as arising from disordered biological mechanisms. The influence of the industry has been present, at least since the 1950s, but with the intensification and broadening of marketing activities, it seems likely that its influence is increasing.

Psychiatric profession

The activities of the pharmaceutical industry may not have been so influential had its message about drugs not suited the interests of the psychiatric profession. Throughout the 20th century the psychiatric profession engaged in a concerted effort to improve its status within society and within medicine. Its strategy was to emphasise the similarity of psychiatry to the rest of medicine. In 1915, the president of the Medico-Psychological Association referred to psychiatry's 'Cinderella' status and to the need for a closer alliance with physical medicine (Editor, 1915).

The enthusiasm for physical treatments of various sorts can be seen as a reflection both of psychiatry's insecurity about its status, and its efforts to improve it. Several historians have argued that physical theories and treatments of madness have always been at the heart of the psychiatric enterprise (Jacyna, 1982; Scull, 1994). Jacyna (1982) has documented how neurophysiological and neuropathological explanations of madness were used to advance the aspirations of psychiatrists in the 19th century and how non-adherence to physicalist explanations was regarded as treachery to the profession. He also demonstrates how 'moral treatment' was opposed by most psychiatrists for its implication that the medically qualified professional was not necessary for successful treatment of the insane. In contrast, other historians have portrayed the history of 20th century psychiatry as the gradual triumph of biologically based psychiatry over fashionable fads such as psychoanalysis (Shorter, 1997). In turn, Scull (1994) has argued that psychoanalysis represents an exception to the general tendency for psychiatry to invoke somatic explanations and treatments for mental disorders and that its influence over mainstream psychiatric thought and practice has been exaggerated.

Empirical evidence from a survey of the most prominent British psychiatric journal of the 20th century supports the idea that there has been a continuous emphasis on biological research and physical treatments with little coverage of psychotherapy, psychoanalysis or social theories or interventions (Moncrieff & Crawford, 2001). Drug research became prominent from the 1950s and has dominated the journal ever since. Other historical research has demonstrated the importance of physical treatments in British and American state hospitals (Moncrieff, 1999; Braslow, 1997; Grob, 1983). Physical treatments, notably electroconvulsive therapy (ECT) and insulin coma therapy, generated enormous enthusiasm within academic psychiatry and hospital settings, and became a central focus of mental hospital activity. Modern drugs appeared to inherit the enthusiasm for these treatment procedures and soon came to be seen as specific rather than symptomatic treatments, again in the mold of the physical treatments (Moncrieff, 1999).

Psychiatry's allegiance to the medical paradigm is also demonstrated by the way in which fashions in psychiatric theory and treatment parallel developments in physical medicine. Thus, at the beginning of the 20th century, when various infectious agents were being discovered, mental disorders were also attributed to chronic infections which lead to the popularity of surgical removal of supposedly infected organs such as teeth and wombs (Grob, 1983). Insulin coma therapy was introduced a few years after the discovery of insulin and at the time of the rise of endocrinology. Modern drugs were introduced shortly after the discovery of penicillin and other antibiotics, which revolutionised the treatment of some infectious diseases.

Another part of the psychiatric profession's strategy to improve its standing was the development of services for more minor psychiatric conditions outside the asylums, which had come to be perceived as increasingly stigmatising due to their isolation and connotations of chronicity. Thus development of acute wards and outpatients services located at general hospitals was advocated (Jones, 1952). Although the neurotic conditions that were increasingly part of such practice, were not always associated with drug treatment, the modelling of psychiatry along the lines of medical services meant that drug treatment could easily be assimilated.

Since the collapse of the albeit modest influence of psychoanalysis and anti-psychiatry, there is little to challenge the hegemony of biological psychiatry. This has also been strengthened by new technology for imaging the brain and the introduction of new classes of drugs. Cognitive behaviour therapy has enjoyed some popularity from among the psychiatric profession as well as elsewhere, but it has never established itself as an alternative to drug treatment except in the mildest of conditions. Despite its popularity among the general public, counselling has been derided by psychiatrists (Wessely, 1996) which is reminiscent of attitudes to moral therapy.

Hence the history of psychiatry reveals that the psychiatric profession has long been wedded to the idea that physical manipulation of body or brain is the correct approach to the treatment of mental disorders. The use of drugs, that 'classic symbolic accoutrement of modern medicine man' (Scull, 1979: 97) has helped the profession to pursue its professional advantage by establishing its medical credentials.

The government

Clive Unsworth (1987) has documented how the government has been the ultimate driving force behind the medicalisation of the treatment of the mad in the United Kingdom since at least the beginning of the 20th century. Policies that advance this position were evident long before the advent of any psychiatric treatments that would currently be considered to be effective. Therefore they demonstrate that the impetus came, not from developments in psychiatry, but from general developments in social policy that became influential from the beginning of the 20th century onwards. These developments are exemplified by Fabianism, and include an acceptance of an increasing role for state intervention, often through the agency of professionals or experts. What had been viewed as moral or political problems came to be defined as technical or scientific ones, that could then be handed over to the correct experts for a solution (Unsworth, 1987). Johnson (1995) has argued that professionals can be seen as being effectively co-opted for the administration of state policy.

In fact government endorsement of medical authority can be traced back to the 1776 Act for the Regulation of Private Madhouses. This introduced the process of certification, which included the obligation for all compulsory admissions to private madhouses to have been examined and 'certified' mad by a medical doctor. However, the 19th century had an ambivalent attitude to the role of medical professionals in psychiatric care and there was some resistance to their increasing involvement (Scull, 1994). Admission to state asylums remained a predominantly legal affair involving a court hearing in which a local magistrate made the decision about compulsory admission.

In the first decades of the 20th century attitudes changed dramatically. By 1924 the MacMillan Commission, which produced the blueprint for the 1930 Mental Treatment Act, boldly stated that 'there is no clear line of demarcation between mental and physical illness' (Royal Commission, 1926). The government and the Commission were critical of the legal nature of the process of compulsory admission and wanted to reduce legal safeguards. They saw this as necessary to increase access to psychiatric treatments and thereby demonstrated their confidence in the benefits of psychiatric intervention. It is interesting to note that minutes of the hearings record that psychiatrists and other representatives of the medical profession were surprised by this confidence in their endeavours (Unsworth, 1987: 211). The Commission did not finally recommend abolition of legal involvement in certification, because of the perceived antagonism of public opinion. However, the Labour government that passed the 1930 Mental Treatment Act further demonstrated its commitment to empowering the psychiatric profession by the fact that it did introduce a treatment order for the admission of some types of patient that did not require the authority of a magistrate.

The 1959 Mental Health Act is usually considered the most medically empowering of psychiatric legislation passed to date. It was this Act that finally dispensed with the involvement of the courts in proceedings concerning compulsory admission to psychiatric hospitals. It enabled such admissions to occur much more informally than before on the basis of two medical recommendations with the approval of a social worker. Again, the Commission and the final Act exceeded the recommendations of the psychiatric and medical profession, who were ambivalent about the wholesale medicalisation of the process of commitment. The Commission, reflecting views within the Ministry of Health, was overwhelmingly convinced about the benign nature and benefits of psychiatric intervention. Therefore treatment was seen as a professional matter that should not come under the remit of an act of Parliament. This was subsequently perceived as one of the main problems of this Act. The Commission's views were probably influenced by the popularity of the physical treatment procedures, and by the early introduction of some of the modern generation of psychotropic drugs (Ewins, 1974).

The 1983 Mental Health Act represents a retrenchment from the trend to medicalise psychiatric legislation, in that it introduced more legal safeguards and placed more restrictions on doctors' powers. It was largely a product of the civil rights and patient advocacy movements of the 1970s. However, since the 1990s, successive governments have again thrown their weight behind increasing medical authority over psychiatric patients, especially the expansion of compulsory powers outside hospital settings. Various measures such as 'supervised discharge' and 'supervision registers' were introduced during the 1990s. One of the principle aims of these measures was to enforce compliance with drug treatment outside hospital. In 1999, the Richardson Committee, set up to make recommendations for new legislation, was told that it must consider how 'the scope of legislation might be extended beyond the hospital to cover care and treatment in community settings' (Department of Health, 1999: 7). The latest draft Mental Health Bill includes provision for compulsory treatment and assessment in the community. Although none of the recent government documents contains a discussion of evidence about the effectiveness and merits of drug treatment, the legislative proposals are based on the assumption that long-term drug treatment will prevent the recurrence of mental disorder and that this is desirable for all parties involved. Hence the new proposals again reflect the willingness of government to adopt an optimistic view of the capabilities of psychiatric interventions. In this instance, this view has helped to justify expanding the remit of compulsory psychiatric powers.

Effects on use and perceptions of drug treatment

The preceding discussion suggests that powerful interests have driven the elevation of psychiatric drug treatments to their current level of prominence. These interests help to promote a certain view of what psychiatric drug treatment aims to achieve and how these drugs are used in practice.

- The view of drugs that is promoted is one that equates them to the use of drugs in other areas of medicine. It relates drug treatment to the correction of chemical imbalances, to which the disorders are attributed. Drugs are viewed as specific treatments and can be contrasted to views of drugs prevalent prior to the 1950s as having essentially symptomatic effects (Moncrieff, 1999). The 'disease centred' model of how psychiatric drugs act is rarely questioned, but there is little evidence to support it (Moncrieff & Cohen, 2005).

- Any debate about the validity of the scientific evidence for the efficacy and utility of psychiatric drugs is potentially skewed. Most academics, researchers, editors, guideline and policy developers are connected with one of the interest groups discussed above. Hence most available material is likely to reflect their interests in promoting the importance and success of drug treatments. Material that suggests otherwise is difficult to publish and publicise.

- Psychiatric drugs are probably over used. Recommendations for cautious and limited prescribing are submerged by the wider impression created by the different interest groups that drugs are the appropriate solution for a widening range of situations.

- The ubiquity of use of psychotropic drugs, and accompanying propaganda, has drawn an ever widening range of human behaviour and distress into a biologically based reductionist explanatory account at the expense of other more complex and sophisticated explanations.

- Non drug based interventions for psychiatric conditions are eclipsed by the prominence of drug treatments.

- The increasing intertwining of psychiatry and drug treatment helps to blur the distinction between medical treatment and social control. Because psychiatric drug treatment appears superficially to be the same activity as the treatment of other medical conditions, and because the administration of drugs is not usually a directly invasive procedure, drug treatment appears as a relatively innocuous process. Contrast this with lobotomy, for example, which is far more easily construed as an act of behavioural manipulation. It is therefore easy to forget that psychotropic drugs are powerful mind altering substances that can also be employed to control and manipulate behaviour.

Alternatives to widespread drugging

Psychiatric drugs have always been a major focus of dissent among the anti-psychiatry movement and the service user movement. They have come to symbolise the dehumanising aspect of psychiatric care. Therefore, since the 1960s there have been attempts to offer care to people with mental disorders that does not revolve around drug treatment. Early experiments included therapeutic communities such as Kingsley Hall and the Arbours Association in the United Kingdom, but these were never systematically evaluated.

During the 1960s and 1970s it was widely recognised in the mainstream psychiatric literature that not all patients benefited from or needed drug treatment, even people with severe psychiatric disorders such as schizophrenia (Carpenter et al, 1977). Long-term follow up of subjects entered into drug trials showed that patients randomised to placebo sometimes had better outcomes (Schooler et al, 1967; Johnstone et al, 1990). This debate however, seems to have been largely forgotten, although some well designed studies suggest that many patients with psychotic breakdowns may be treatable without the use of antipsychotic drugs.

In the 1970s, Loren Mosher, a psychiatrist, set up the Soteria project in the United States. This consisted of a small residential unit staffed largely by non professionals with a philosophy of providing low key empathic care and minimising the use of drug treatment, especially antipsychotic drugs. From the beginning he evaluated the success of the project through a randomised trial comparing it to usual hospital based care. Successive potential admissions with early onset schizophrenia were admitted by random allocation either to Soteria or to the local psychiatric hospital. In an early evaluation of the first six weeks of care based on 100 patients, 67 per cent of Soteria treated patients had not had any drug treatment compared with none of the control patients. Only 12 per cent of the Soteria group had had continuous drug treatment compared with 98 per cent of the controls (Mosher et al, 1995). At two year follow up 42 per cent of Soteria patients had been drug free throughout compared with 3 per cent of hospital treated patients. Only 19 per cent of Soteria patients had received continuous drug treatment (Bola & Mosher, 2003). Two year outcome data from 160 patients showed that Soteria treated patients had very similar outcomes to the conventionally treated group, with some possible areas of superiority such as fewer readmissions and more living alone. However the length of stay in the Soteria project was considerably longer at 129 days.

There were also some other problems with the Soteria project. Numerous outcome measures were used and very complex analysis was employed, so it is not easy to make direct comparisons between the groups. Also some reports exclude people who dropped out of the Soteria project before 28 days, which would remove some of the people who would be considered to be failures for the Soteria project. However, despite these drawbacks the project suggests that a substantial proportion of patients with early onset schizophrenia can be cared for without the use of antipsychotic drugs and achieve a comparable outcome to those who are prescribed these drugs.

This conclusion is supported by another recent project conducted in Finland. This study compared patients treated by teams with a philosophy of minimal use of neuroleptic drugs with patients treated with good standard usual care (Lehtinen et al, 2000).

As shown in Table 7.1, 43 per cent of people treated by the teams with the minimal neuroleptic use philosophy did not receive these drugs at all compared with 6 per cent of the comparison group. Two year outcomes were slightly, but convincingly, better for the minimal use group. They spent less time in hospital, had fewer psychotic symptoms and better global functioning. These results were strengthened after controlling for age, gender and diagnosis.

Table 7.1   Results of the Finnish Minimal Use Study

Outcome	Minimal use	Control	Total	p[a] value
Used no neuroleptic drugs	43%	6%		<0.001
Less than 2weeks in hospital	51%	26%	42%	0.01
No psychotic symptoms in past yr	58%	41%	52%	0.09
Employed	33%	31%	32%	0.80
GAS[b] score 7 or more	49%	25%	40%	0.02

[a] p value is the probability that this result would occur by chance. Conventionally p < 0.05 is taken to indicate that the result shows a true association

[b] GAS = Global Assessment Scale

The two studies described above, and other similar studies (Carpenter et al, 1977; Ciompi et al, 1993) indicate that a substantial proportion of people with early onset psychosis do well without the use of standard drug treatment, and point towards possibilities for reducing psychiatry's reliance on drugs. Unfortunately, institutional psychiatry has taken little notice of these results.

Conclusions

The question at the heart of this discussion is whether psychiatric drugs have risen to their current prominent position in psychiatry and elsewhere solely as a consequence of their intrinsic merits, or whether external influences have helped to create this situation. A brief critique of the evidence base suggests that the benefits of psychiatric drugs in many situations are debatable. In particular there are questions about the benefits of the use of long-term drug treatment in schizophrenia and other psychotic disorders and manic depression. There are questions about the utility of antidepressants for both acute and long-term treatment. And evidence that many people with severe psychiatric conditions can be treated without drugs has been neglected.

The reason that the deficiencies in the evidence have gone largely unremarked may be due to the fact that three powerful institutions have had an interest in promoting psychiatric drug treatments and the medical and biological paradigms that usually justify and inform their use. In the case of the pharmaceutical industry and the psychiatric profession the promotion of drug treatment appears to have advanced financial interests and professional ambitions. In the government's case, the promotion of drug treatment is related to long-standing political policies that transformed social and legal problems into scientific and technical ones. In psychiatry this was seen in the transfer of authority for compulsion from the legal apparatus of the state to the medical profession, which has been accompanied by an expansion of the possible application of compulsory powers.

The power of the institutions involved, and their virtual monopoly on the production of publicly available and officially sanctioned information, means that it is difficult to discuss the potential harms involved in the overselling of drugs. It is also difficult to formulate alternative approaches to drug treatment itself, approaches which might emphasise the non specific effects of drugs and more patient centred evaluation of drug effects (Moncrieff & Cohen, 2005). Where people have managed to run treatment projects that attempt to minimise drug use these have generally been successful. But the psychiatric community appears to have lost the ability to imagine that life with serious mental illness is possible, and maybe sometimes better, without drugs; that psychiatric drugs may be a short-term necessity in some cases but are not a solution to the complex problems of living that are currently labelled as psychiatric disorders.

8

British Mental Health Social Work and the Psychosocial Approach in Context

Shulamit Ramon

This chapter looks at the options and dilemmas facing British mental health social workers in the 21st century in the light of their past and present. The discussion is placed in on the one hand the context of the psychosocial approach to mental health (Ramon & Williams, 2005). On the other hand it is also focused on understanding the dynamics of a welfare bureaucracy profession, impacted by political changes at both central and local government levels, which has encouraged an increasing belief in the value of managerialism as against psychosocial professionalism. An account of the impact of this duality on the profession is necessary to understand the role and contribution of social work in mental health, as well as its shortcomings and dilemmas. A further duality is located within the social work profession, which is less well established than the older professions of medicine and law, at times called a 'semi-profession' (Toren, 1972), by its anchor in a value system focused on the right of troubled individuals to respect, self-determination and social support, yet with a social mandate which includes both care and control.

Social workers and most mental health professions (with the exception of psychologists) share a largely anti-theoretical stance, which entails perceiving educators and researchers as divorced from practice, and practitioners and managers as viewing conceptual frameworks to be unnecessary. Knowledge of research and implementation of research findings continue to be relatively rare among practitioners, although the establishment at the end of 2001 of the Social Care Institute for Excellence (SCIE) and a new social care inspectorate in 2004 focusing its work on the evidence base of social work, signify attempts to disseminate research and give it a higher profile. Educators argue that their role is to ensure that students need to be prepared for best available practice as well as improving it, rather than for the run of the mill workplace. However, employers seem to prefer workers who do as they are told, and are ready for whatever they may find in practice. The strong anti-theoretical stance held by both employers and most practitioners also militates against the reflective thinking which would help practitioners and managers to offer more in-depth work, a cornerstone of the psychosocial approach to social work in general as much as to mental health in particular (Scohn, 1987; Yelloly & Henkel, 1995).

The chapter looks mainly at options and dilemmas in the context of working with adults experiencing mental health problems, yet a large number of the issues raised also relate to mental health social work with children and adolescents (Walker, 2003).

Mental health social work (MHSW) – a contextualised and multifaceted profession

British MHSW began in 1920, when the first social worker was appointed to the Tavistock clinic; the second such appointment took place only in 1927, to the Jewish child guidance clinic in Hackney (Timms, 1964). Traditionally social workers followed a psychosocial model of mental health and illness. This was reflected in their preference for a loose psychodynamic approach to mental illness, a strong belief in non-institutionalised and non-medicalised interventions of both a psychological and social nature (Timms, 1964). They took for granted the connections between poverty, social deprivation and mental illness, and accepted by and large the critique put forward by the anti-psychiatry movement in the 1960s and 70s. Most mental health social workers believed that users were over-medicated, and had doubts concerning the validity of psychiatric diagnosis.

Since the late 1980s, social workers have been influenced by (i) the social role valorisation (SRV) approach and (ii) by lessons learned from child abuse.

Social role valorisation

The SRV perspective originated in Scandinavia in the 1950s in rehabilitation work with people with learning disabilities. It was publicised in the 1960s and later in North America by Wolf Wolfsenberger from the institute of Mental Retardation in Toronto (Nirje, 1969; Wolfsenberger, 1972, 1983). Its protagonists argue that the Western approach to people with disabilities has generalised the disability into the totality of the person, thus creating stereotyped caricatures which inhibit these people from having the ordinary life they deserve like everybody else. However, unlike Goffman (1961, 1969) – the originator of the theoretical and experiential understanding of stigma – SRV believes it is possible to reverse the impact of stigma, and thus enable people with disabilities to lead a more ordinary life than was the case in the last two hundred years since the creation of total institutions (Ramon, 1991).

For such a change to take place, professionals, lay people, and disabled people themselves need to change their attitudes towards the disability and its carriers, as well as provide concrete opportunities in which they can create a better life for themselves. Thus SRV is a mixture of a sociopsychological framework, together with a pragmatic emphasis on service re-organisation coming clearly from an ideology of inclusive citizenship. SRV captured the imagination of some disabled people, and coincided with the development of a social model of disability by themselves (Swain et al, 1996), as well as the imagination of social workers, some psychologists, and some policy makers. Very few doctors were convinced by it, and Wolfensberger's view of mental health professionals has been particularly negative, because he saw them as continuing to perpetuate a pathological perspective of their clients (Wolfensberger, 1989).

The approach matched well the attempt to de-institutionalise the variety of total institutions in the UK in the 1980s, which is when SRV came to the knowledge of British professionals. SRV became an ideal to strive towards rather than an everyday practice for most social workers, because of the bureaucratic structures in which they worked and the conformity to the traditional pathology model by most directors of health and social care services for all disabled people.

The awareness of child abuse

The lessons from the discovery of child abuse, and in particular of sexual abuse, have been very different. These focused on a high level of empathy with the victim, and the deep-seated trauma s/he has suffered, which is difficult to shake off and likely to have long-term effects, of which experiencing mental ill health is a distinct possibility (Williams, 2005).

Old (psychoanalysis) and new (eg. dialectic behavioural therapy) therapeutic interventions have been applied to the work with victims of abuse, with the recognition of the effect of this type of work not only on the client, but also on the therapist. Little understanding has been attempted in relation to the perpetrator (often the father, a step father or mum's boyfriend) and to the other parent (usually the mother), often accused of colluding with the perpetrator. An interesting conceptual and practice oriented social work approach was taken by Mullender & Ward (1991). They undertook self-directed groupwork with mothers whose children had been abused, focusing on empowering them to be an advocacy group for themselves and their children, as well as to work on the very complex and difficult feelings the abuse had made them experience, concerning themselves, the abusive ex-partner and the abused child.

The focus on the abused child has led to a diminished interest in the adult client with mental illness in favour of working with neglected and abused children, and to building a reputation among women users of mental health service of social work as a profession which is there to take away one's children.

Other conceptual innovations

Thus historically the social work perspective offered a contextualised and multifaceted approach to mental ill health. Today too, while most social workers would not deny the value of medical input in the field of mental health, they perceive it as a narrow and insufficient perspective, and would prefer mental health services to be dominated by a broad psychosocial framework.

The focus on a contextualised, psychosocial and empowering, non-biomedical, approach is highlighted in a number of conceptual and practice innovations closely related to a social work value base since the 1960s. These include:

a   Paying attention to institutional abuse, child and elder abuse, and the strong connection between abuse and mental ill health (Stanley, Manthorpe & Penhale, 1999). While the conceptual and analytic interest in institutions came initially from sociology, especially medical sociology, the focus on institutional abuse and its analysis in terms of the impact on different clients and service givers developed within social work. It highlights the interaction between organisational structures and their users, as well as between these structures and their employees, in meeting the specific social mandate institutions have at a given historical period. The anti-institutionalism stance is also closely connected to the focus in social work on care in the community and networking (Trevillion, 1992), though the conceptual aspect of this position was developed more in sociology and social policy (Bulmer, 1987).

b   Self-directed groupwork highlighting the possibility of putting together community development with empowerment principles (Mullender & Ward, 1991). The example of groupwork with mothers of abused children outlined above illustrates well the focus of this approach on troubled, vulnerable and oppressed minorities who nevertheless have in the view of the social worker the ability to be empowered and to use it positively to enhance the quality of their own lives, those of their children, and the community in which they live. It also demonstrates the attempt to conceptualise and introduce change beyond the individual and her family.

c   An emphasis on partnership working with users, and their involvement in policy making, training and research (Barnes & Bowl, 2001; Castillo, 2003; Ramon, 2003; Beresford, 2005). This has been a core component of social work education since the 1990s, while remaining less applied in practice. It is linked to the contribution of SRV and the newly emerging focus on citizenship and participation (Beresford & Croft, 1993; Bray & Preston-Shoot, 1995).

d   Anti-discrimination in its implications for ethnic minorities, disabled people, women and poor people. This has been a much more pronounced feature of training in social work than in any other helping profession. This emphasis relates to the value put on the right of the individual to a dignified life free from oppression, and an entitlement to civil rights regardless of origin. It also entails an analysis of the underlying factors leading to discrimination and its maintenance.

MHSW – a tradition of innovatory practice

The above conceptual innovations were reflected in practice innovations too, such as:

a   Establishing attachments of social workers to primary care, beginning in a Kentish Town practice in 1966. Social workers offered counselling and benefits advice, a typical psychosocial mix not provided by any other profession. Although this attachment was judged as successful by social workers, service users, GPs and psychiatrists (Brewer & Lait, 1978), local authorities withdraw social workers from primary care in the early 80s, as this initiative was not obligatory. Today too, while we are witnessing a wider professional mix within primary care, social workers continue to be generally excluded.

b   The Barnet Intensive Crisis Intervention Service, pioneered by social workers and psychiatrists in 1974, one of the few holistic services focused on minimising the use of hospitalisation that existed in this country for a long time. This service provides a rapid response to crisis from a multidisciplinary team, often in people's home, including an exploration of non-hospital alternatives to the resolution of the crisis. The conceptual approach underpinning the Barnet service highlights the interdependency within a family system where the identified client expresses the family dilemma and his expulsion from the family through hospitalisation enables the others to attempt to 'break clean'. The intervention on offer tries to prevent the expulsion and to treat instead the problem at the core of the family dynamic. The team also uses biofeedback and environmental interventions, thus offering a truly biopsychosocial model. While research evidence has amply demonstrated the effectiveness of this service (Barnes et al, 1990; Mitchell, 1993), it did not become a beacon service to be followed, due to the threat it presented to traditional psychiatry. Although the contribution of social workers to initiating the service and to its theoretical development has been well documented by Mitchell (1993), this fact is hardly remembered or recognised within MHSW and the multidisciplinary community in general.

c   Social workers at the Family Welfare Association in Tower Hamlet – influenced and supported by the sociologist George Brown (Brown & Harris, 1978) – who initiated a project in which isolated mothers became members of groups led by local women in their homes in the early 70s. The organisation provided training, supervision, a budget for refreshments, and a very modest pay to the group leaders. The project was evaluated to be a success, but was discontinued when the political climate changed (Knight, 1978). It took a more community orientated, social capital building and mutual support approach than the innovations outlined above. Its initiators believed that the community can have its own home grown leaders, and that these informal leaders can sufficiently befriend and enable isolated mothers to get out of the cycle of depression and isolation, not only to invest in mutual support of each other, but also to venture further into finding themselves a socially valued role beside motherhood.

d   The Chesterfield Support Network, established by Derbyshire social services in 1982, a model of user-run large group and some satellite groups, as well as an individualised advisory service provided by social workers, based in an ordinary community centre used by more than twenty community groups (Hennelly, 1990). This approach is based not only on a community work model, but also on belief in the ability of hitherto vulnerable service users to support each other, to largely manage their own groups, without necessarily stopping to experience mental ill health. Established sometime before the discovery of the concept of recovery, this project highlights the strengths of combining individual casework with group and community work in a context in which SRV is practised as a tool in enabling recovery, when the latter is defined as taking control over one's life (Wallcraft, 2005).

e   The first user policy forum in the UK – the Camden Consortium – established by Iris Nutting, then team leader of Camden social services in Friern Barnet hospital in North London (1984). A number of its members have become leaders of the British user movement. The forum provided an early example of the abilities of mental health service users, including the capacity to work in a disciplined way within a group over a lengthy period of time, as long as they are assured of being entrusted to carry out this important piece of work. This project is a good example of SRV, involvement and participation in everyday practice.

f   Social workers initiating and leading the development of the Building Bridges project, which attended to the needs of parents with mental illness and their children in different, and imaginative ways (Diggins, 2000). This project, initiated locally in Lewisham, has expanded today into nine such specialised services as well as into a national network titled Parental Mental Health and Children Network, based at SCIE (the Social Care Institute of Excellence), aimed at promoting better practices at this interface between adults and children (see ScieDrive, the network newsletter, of February 2005). It illustrates a psychosocial approach and a holistic one to the family, where 'holistic' means paying attention to the differential needs of each family member, as well as to those of the family unit.

The Approved Social Worker (ASW) era

Social work is clearly impacted by political decisions and ideological shifts of politicians leading central and local government. Until the 1980s social work attempted to maintain a focus on individuals (casework), as well as on groups and communities (groupwork and community work), though only a few workers combined both approaches in their everyday practice.

The ascent of the Conservative government to power in 1979 meant the destruction of community work as an integral part of social work. The entry of Labour to power in 1997 was reflected in the re-establishment of community development approaches, exemplified in the government's flagship programme Sure Start, though without reinclusion within social work.

A third year has been added to the basic qualification of social workers, and post-qualifying training is required for those working in mental health and child care by the Labour government. At the same time a more punitive approach to offenders meant that training for the probation service has been taken out of social work education by the same Labour government, continuing the wish of the previous government. The managerial ethos which began under the Conservative government continues to be adhered to by the Labour government too.

Negative attitudes towards local authorities and the gradual erosion in their powers by both successive Conservative and Labour governments, have also impacted on reducing the power of social work. The relocation of mental health social workers into Mental Health Partnership Trusts is too new to know its full effects (Department of Health, 2004a), but the anecdotal evidence highlights that most of the 4225 social workers thus attached feel threatened by it as it turned them into a minority group within a medically dominated service (Huxley et al, 2004).

Social work has been perceived as too soft by successive governments, an issue compounded by the growing focus on risk avoidance (Foster, 2005). While the focus on risk avoidance dates to the early 1990s, the current post 9/11/2001 political climate reinforces it and prevents a proper re-appraisal of our risk policy in mental health.

The most central change in MHSW since the postwar years has been the introduction of the Approved Social Work (ASW) in the mental health system, a role legislated through the 1983 Amendments to the Mental Health Act. The role requires assessing the need for compulsory admission on the basis of risk analysis and following-up such an admission, while looking for the least restrictive alternatives to hospitalisation, and working closely with family members in certain circumstances. It enables social workers an autonomous position vis-à-vis other assessors, notably psychiatrists and GPs (Barnes et al, 1990).

From the legislator's perspective social workers replaced relatives in this highly complex role, expected to offer a psychosocial perspective to balance the biomedical model brought in by the psychiatrists and GPs. Carrying out such an assessment at the point of intense crisis calls for well developed skills of assessment of a variety of risks and resources, thorough knowledge of the law, mental health and community resources, as well as a sensitive approach to users and their family members. Thus the role exists within the interface of risk avoidance, maintaining human rights and a psychosocial stance within a crisis context.

However, several obstacles to meeting the role requirements have emerged. These include:

a   The tools necessary for psychosocial work – as distinct from psychosocial assessment – were not (and still are not) there in the first place. The development of less restrictive alternative settings in which people could be looked after in a mental health crisis has been patchy and unsatisfactory in the country as a whole, thus disabling ASWs from fulfilling their obligation in this respect. Insufficient time has been allocated to follow up work, while time is a major component in building up a trusting working relationship between workers, clients and their relatives, following a major trauma such as a psychiatric crisis ending in a hospital admission.

b   The increasing focus on risk assessment since the early 1990s has led to a further erosion of the psychosocial dimension in the assessment process. This has meant that only risk *avoidance* has/is been focused upon, at the expense of risk *taking* (Ramon, 2005). It is not possible to work successfully with service users without them having challenges to strive towards, and these entail risk taking, albeit in a calculated risk assessment framework. As a result, a psychosocial approach to risk has hardly been developed or applied in practice.

c   The ever-present tension within social work between care and control has been tilted significantly in ASW work towards the control end of the range. This means that social workers not wishing to concentrate on controlling tasks do not enter mental health, and those remaining find themselves doing more control work and less care work. Carrying out control work in a partnership and demonstrating respect to clients is extremely challenging. While ASW training does highlight some of these issues, the working environment rarely encourages it.

d   Low morale among existing ASW, coupled by low rate of recruitment of new ones has been reported in a recent study of the Social Care Workforce Research Unit (Huxley et al, 2003). Most ASWs are not aware of the history of conceptual and practice innovations outlined above.

e   The lack of sufficient numbers of ASWs and MHSWs, coupled with the legal obligation of local authorities to provide ASW cover, had led to curtailing most of the work which was not directly legislated for in the Mental Health Act, such as:
-   family work;
-   group work;
-   work with people who had mild mental health problems;
-   any type of preventive work.

Social workers wishing to continue the above areas of work in a significant way have to battle with their managers, find alternative sources of funding which would free them from the ASW rota for a while, move to part-time work as ASW while working elsewhere on what they believe to be essential psychosocial mental health work, or move to work in the voluntary sector.

f Recovery (Wallcraft, 2005), social inclusion (Mind, 1999; Morris, 2004) and a focus on the existential needs of users (Wagner & King, 2005) are yet to make a difference to the way ASWs are trained and how they practice. Although these developments fit well within a broad psychosocial approach, their implementation requires not only an attitudinal shift within and beyond the mental health system, but also a re-positioning of the working partnership with users and informal carers, and investment in working with the wider social environment.

Although social workers were initially doubtful about becoming ASWs due to its clear controlling (and potentially coercive) aspect, the role has brought them prestige within the multidisciplinary context of mental health work, higher pay, and some autonomy as it enabled them to oppose recommendations for compulsory admission when in disagreement with psychiatrists and GPs (Barnes et al, 1990). All of this is seductive for a profession often treated as an outsider by the rest of the mental health system.

To become an ASW, social workers who have already been in practice for two years following their qualification have to undertake a 60 days training programme, followed by five days updating training per year. Performance is assessed by practice teachers and through written assignments. This needs to be compared to the two days mandatory training for psychiatrists, and ten days for GPs. ASW training is provided by local consortia, some of which are linked to universities and some are not, regulated and monitored by the Central Council of Education and Training in Social Work (CCETSW) until 2002, replaced now by the General Council of Social Care (GCSC).

Training is offered as a mixture of lectures, seminars and supervised practice, in which 120 competencies have to be mastered. Yet crucial elements are often missing from this package, such as actively searching for the least restrictive alternative to hospitalisation, methods of working with the Nearest Relative and other family members and friends (Rapaport, 2005), advocacy and user empowerment, and effecting social inclusion.

By now all ASW courses involve service users and carers as trainers, and some also involve them as learners. Likewise, most mental health training modules on the basic qualification for social work engage users and relatives in the training, and place students for supervised fieldwork in user-run organisations. This type of systematic involvement – which can be tokenistic at times, but does not have to be so – is yet to happen in other mental health professions.

MHSW involvement in policy and structural changes

As already mentioned social work has been treated as a marginalised professional group by successive governments in part due to its location within local authorities, and in part due to its liberal, 'soft' image. Perhaps its focus on a complex approach, which the psychosocial perspective requires, has added to it being mistrusted by central government. Social work has also been marginalised within the mental health system which was/is dominated by a medicalised approach to mental illness and health and which at best has an ambivalent response to psychosocial approaches, if not an outright negative one.

This attitude is reflected in the role allocated to MHSWs in major policy initiatives, such as the psychiatric hospitals closure programme and the development of community mental health teams. Social workers have been the only professional group to be fully committed to care in the community since the 50s (Ramon, 1985). Although more knowledgeable about communities and care in the community than other mental health profession, they were largely excluded from having an active role in the hospitals closure and resettlement programme, due to the wish of the health sector to retain control of this programme. In some cases social workers felt scapegoated by other staff in the hospitals during the closure process, in retribution for their support of the closure (Ramon, 1992).

Social workers involved in resettlement work have been portrayed by the media as callous and stupid (Wallace, 1985). Social workers looked forward to community mental health teams collaboration, but also with trepidation to being led by psychiatrists and losing their autonomy in the process. The current co-existence of social workers with community mental health nurses, where leadership of the joint teams alternates and in which psychiatrists are marginalised, makes social workers happier but also wary of the possibility that nurses will take over traditional social work functions. Nurses in the community mental health teams have in fact adopted and implemented some typical social work responses, albeit invariably without acknowledging that this is the case. Psychiatrists focusing on open supported employment are sure they have invented the strengths approach, which in fact originated in North American social work in the late 1980s and the early 1990s (Saleeby, 1992).

The verdict is out as to whether collaboration has in fact improved, especially between social workers and health workers, and whether these teams simply pander to 'the lowest common denominator', namely the medical model (Galvin & McCarthy, 1994; Onyett & Ford, 1996). It is also unclear as to whether the mergers of mental health NHS trusts with Social Services teams as from April 2001 have changed much the character of the collaboration. Judging from the Northern Ireland experience of unified health and social care services, social workers stand to lose in autonomy, with no visible gains to either MHSWs or to service users (Campbell, 1998). Will the current disappearance of social services departments as we know them curtail further the professional autonomy of social workers?

The introduction of care management, and later of the care programme approach (CPA) in mental health has added on the one hand more co-ordinating, managerial tasks to the workforce, as well as some opportunities to match services to needs rather than vice versa. Most MHSWs felt it took away from them further the possibility of therapeutic encounters with clients, but gave them some power to impact care packages. However, the transfer of the overall responsibility for care management from social workers to psychiatrists in 1995 in the wake of a periodical media scandal about killings by mentally ill people, even though the first group has had a lot more experience of care management, highlighted further the marginality of MHSWs.

The British Association of Social Workers (BASW) leadership is committed to supporting good psychosocial practice. The organisation has a relatively active special interest group on mental health, responding regularly to policy proposals and sending representatives to various collaborative bodies (eg. the Mental Health Alliance). However, unlike its stance in the 70s and 80s, most of its activities have not been proactive, and the group represents only a minority of those working in this branch of the profession.

Despite its justified credentials for being pro-users, the BASW mental health special interest group has not initially rebelled against the government's draconian policy towards people with anti-social personality disorder. Social workers based in forensic settings have created their own special interest group, reflecting the view that their interests and concerns are apart from the rest of MHSWs. By now, in 2006, BASW is part of the Mental Health Alliance which strongly opposes this measure in the proposed new Mental Health Act.

The recent focus on mental health promotion and prevention in the context of – social inclusion (see Standard 1 of the National Service Framework for Mental Health, Department of Health, 1998b) – in which psychosocial factors have a more prominent place – is yet to make its impact on MHSWs or on their policy advisory groups.

Only one director of social services, but no frontline social worker, was a member of the Expert Committee advising the government on desirable changes in the 1983 Mental Health Act. She has campaigned vigorously for the adoption of the committee's recommendations.

A window of opportunity? The future role and contribution of mental health social work

The Expert Committee chaired by Generva Richardson (Department of Health, 1999) recommended that not only social workers will carry out the work currently performed by ASWs. This recommendation has been met with concern and opposition among MHSWs. Some of these sentiments have to do with fears of loss of power and prestige; some with acknowledging that no other profession has the training necessary for providing a psychosocial perspective necessary within compulsory admission work.

I share the second concern, as the largest group of professionals in mental health services – nurses – would need a lot more than the current 60 days of training to become an ASW to adopt the knowledge, attitudes and values necessary for applying a psychosocial approach. Nurses would need to be trained by social workers and shadow them in their daily work if indeed they were to follow a psychosocial approach in their assessments.

However, MHSWs should seriously consider that not having the sole responsibility for ASW work would free social workers to use their knowledge and skills more broadly in working with users and their families. This would be more beneficial to users, relatives, social workers, and mental health services in general, as it will bring its psychosocial perspective to the fore. It would constitute one step further towards the active reduction of the dominance of the biomedical model in these services by promoting a competing, yet potentially complimentary, model of values, theory and practice.

Existing models of practice of MHSW have been insufficiently influenced by newer and more promising directions of conceptual and practice developments of psychosocial approaches, which include:

- the strengths approach – outlined above – which was developed within social work in the early 90s and most social work students would have been taught something about it, although it is not applied in everyday practice (Rapp, 1992). It is closely related to the focus on social capital and capacity building (Wilkinson, 1996), yet both concepts are hardly explored in MHSW (or in social work in general and throughout the mental health system) and rarely applied in its practice;

- the convincing argument from the protagonists of the social disability model that disability per se is not a sufficient barrier to having a valued place in society or leading a life of good quality. The able-bodied have created a society which prevents the acceptance of those disabled (Swain et al, 1996). The systematic application of this model to mental ill health, and to MHSW, is yet to happen despite the noted impact of SRV on social work.
- the strong focus in social work theory and in social work education on structural barriers to the participation of service users as valued citizens, which has insufficiently permeated MHSW practice, even though it pioneered such participation.
- knowledge and use in everyday practice of brief and focused therapeutic interventions (eg. cognitive behavioural therapy, psychosocial interventions, solution focused therapy).

The reconstruction of the psychosocial approach needs to take these areas into consideration. Given this background, MHSWs need to ask themselves where their unique contribution to the field of mental health lies; and how the re-building of a comprehensive psychosocial approach spanning theory, policy, practice and research can be enhanced.

Renewed evidence indicates that it is the quality of the interaction between the individual and the social context which is crucial for their well-being (Glouberman, 2001; Duggan, 2002b). This re-emphasises the importance of holding to the connections between the psychological and the social, rather than opting for the recent fashion which discards the 'psycho' in favour of the 'social' or vice versa.

The above indicates that MHSW has a lot to offer to the re-construction of such an approach, but only if this comes with a thorough re-appraisal of the past, moving away from defensive positions, finding allies to work with in this process, rather than waiting for others to take the initiative, forging a new identity and constructing a context more conducive to psychosocial work.

Conclusion

To summarise, for most of the period between 1983 and 2000 mental health social workers with adults have been engaged in the process of compulsory admission, risk assessment and avoidance, care management and the Care Programme Approach (CPA), ensuring that users got their benefits in a system that has not become simpler or easier to work with, and some counselling and some joint work with their colleagues in child protection.

Those working in child and family consultation services focused mostly on child protection issues and the arrest and prevention of abuse. Domestic violence – an area of major innovation led by social workers – has not been part of the agenda of MHSWs; nor have employment and education become part of everyday work with clients. Most MHSWs are not currently engaged in any user-led activity, group work or community work; the same applies to preventive work, including such work with mothers who suffer from mental illness, even though this group represents a major component of their caseload. The involvement in legal work – in mental health and in child protection – brought a clear focus and social-professional recognition to mental health social work. The question is at what cost, and whether this is where MHSWs would like to remain in the 21st century.

It seems to me that in terms of the values social work stands for, its past contribution, and the useful potential contribution it can offer service users, carers, and our society, as well as enabling greater professional satisfaction, MHSW would need to broaden its mandate and move beyond the role of the ASW to a more full-scale psychosocial practice.

A number of changes which have taken place towards the end of the 20th century have brought the psychosocial approach to mental health to the fore. These include:

- the closure of most of our psychiatric hospital and the resettlement of the long-stay patients in the community
- the focus of mental health services work has shifted from cure to care
- greater, and more focused, recognition of the limitations of the medical approach in the field of mental health (Breggin, 1985; Rogers & Pilgrim, 2001; Bracken & Thomas, 2001; Bentall, 2003; Double, 2005a)
- the prevention of social exclusion and the promotion of social inclusion are socially and politically accepted as essential parameters which impact on service users, but are yet to impact on everyday professional input
- the work carried out by nurses and social workers is becoming more similar in several aspects
- users are more heard and some are more involved in providing an input into service planning, training and research; as well as in running alternative services (Barnes & Bowl, 2001; Sedley, 2000; Ramon, 2003), yet working in a more equal partnership with users is yet to be developed within mainstream psychiatry and MHSW
- carers have a formal right to being assessed as to their own needs; their views are more taken into account by professionals; they have a

stronger voice and are more provided with support groups and educational opportunities (Rapaport, 2005)

- a much greater emphasis on creating educational and employment opportunities for service users can be observed (Perkins et al, 1997; Secker et al, 2002)
- more and better developed advocacy, direct payment, user and carer networking schemes have become available to service users and carers
- the range of brief psychosocial therapeutic intervention has been enlarged, but is not yet part of the repertoire of MHSWs.

While these shifts have highlighted the need for a solid psychosocial approach, MHSWs, alongside the other stakeholders in mental health, need to consider the following questions:

- Has the role of the ASW provided what it was supposed to offer?
- What has been the cost to users, carers, social workers and other members of the multidisciplinary team of the nearly exclusive focus in MHSW on ASW work?
- What should be the reformulated psychosocial approach, one which takes into account the changes outlined above in values, concepts, issues, knowledge, skills, and modes of practice, and the perspectives of different stakeholders?
- How are we going to achieve a mental health system impacted by psychosocial approaches, including the identification of the barriers and opportunities on the way to this achievement?

9

Democracy, Citizenship and the Radical Possibilities of Postpsychiatry

Pat Bracken & Philip Thomas

Introduction

The 20th century is often held up as the great era of democracy. It was a time of struggles and successes. Women won the right to vote for the first time in many countries and colonial rule came to an end in different parts of the world. But democracy is about something greater than politics and parliaments – it concerns ordinary people having control of their lives. This is a wider issue than who is allowed to vote, when, where and for whom.

When it comes to controlling our own lives and destinies it is clear that in the past 50 years various forms of technology have dominated how we work, how we communicate with one another, how we travel and what we do with our leisure, in short how we live our lives. But technology is not restricted to machines and gadgets, computers and mobile phones; it also concerns systems of knowledge and expertise. It concerns how we order our reality and, increasingly, our relationships.

Arguably one of the greatest expansions of technology in recent years has been in the world of mental health. At the beginning of the 21st century we have a huge (and growing) pharmaceutical industry, one branch of which is dedicated to the production of various chemicals to regulate our thoughts and emotions. We have an array of machines to scan our brains for different types of activity. But the technology of psychiatry has expanded in other directions as well. Alongside psychodynamic therapies we have cognitive-behavioural therapies and different systems of family intervention. There are psychosocial interventions for schizophrenia, numerous 'tools' to assess personality, motivation and compliance and of course to assess 'risk'.

If democracy concerns ordinary people controlling their lives, questions arise about who controls and shapes the nature of this technology. What assumptions guide the theories and practice of psychiatry and its associated therapies? Are these assumptions valid? Could we, and should we, work with different assumptions, with different priorities? Our argument is that the struggle for democracy did not end with the demolition of the Berlin wall. Neither, for that matter, will it end after the so-called war on terror. It is very much alive today in the field of mental health, and will continue long into the future. It is time now for an open and democratic debate about mental health. At present we have a very limited debate about what is helpful and of value when we experience madness and distress. The parameters of this debate are set largely by corporate (mainly pharmaceutical) and professional (mainly psychiatric) interests.

Postpsychiatry is about creating spaces in which voices customarily excluded from this debate can participate. In this chapter, we shall discuss the key guiding assumptions of 20th century psychiatry, and then point out reasons why these assumptions need to be challenged. We then consider the radical possibilities of postpsychiatry with reference to the liberatory activities of groups like Mad Pride. We end by looking at the idea of citizenship from a number of points of view.

Modernist psychiatry

Both critics and supporters agree that, historically, modern psychiatry is a product of the European Enlightenment. Prior to the Enlightenment, or the Age of Reason as it is also called, the concept of mental illness as a separate area of medical endeavour simply did not exist; there were no psychiatrists or psychiatric patients as such. It is only with the intellectual and cultural developments of the Age of Reason that we see a field of medical work open up which eventually becomes psychiatry.

The Age of Reason is difficult to define and to locate historically. However, beginning in the mid-17th century there was a major shift in European culture. It is impossible to say exactly why the Enlightenment began and why it developed as it did. Some historians argue that it began with the rise of science, others with the rise of capitalism. Other factors were the emerging bureaucracy in most European states and the fact of colonialism and increasing literacy. However, these influences weren't unidirectional, the assumptions which were at stake in the Enlightenment also fed into these developments.

Enlightenment meant a turn towards the light, the light of reason. This meant turning away from religious revelation and the wisdom of the ancient world towards science and rationality as the path towards truth and progress. In practical terms, the Enlightenment spawned an era in which society sought to rid itself of all 'unreasonable' elements. As the historian Roy Porter writes:

> And the enterprise of the age of reason, gaining authority from the mid-17th century onwards, was to criticise, condemn and crush whatever its protagonists considered to be foolish or unreasonable. All beliefs and practices which appeared ignorant, primitive, childish or useless came to be readily dismissed as idiotic or insane, evidently the products of stupid thought-processes, or delusion and daydream. And all that was so labelled could be deemed inimical to society or the state – indeed could be regarded as a menace to the proper workings of an orderly, efficient, progressive, rational society.
>
> Porter, 1987: 14-15

According to Michel Foucault (1967), the emergence of the institutions in which 'unreasonable' people were to be housed was not in itself a 'progressive', or medical, venture. It was simply, and crudely, an act of social exclusion which he described as 'The great confinement'. Furthermore, he argued that it was only when such people had been both excluded and brought together that they became subject to the 'gaze' of medicine. According to Foucault, Porter and other historians, doctors were originally involved in these institutions in order to treat physical illness and to offer moral guidance. They were not there as experts in disorders of the mind. As time went on, the medical profession came to dominate in these institutions and doctors began to order and classify the inmates in more systematic ways. Roy Porter writes:

> Indeed, the rise of psychological medicine was more the consequence than the cause of the rise of the insane asylum. Psychiatry could flourish once, but not before, large numbers of inmates were crowded into asylums.
>
> Porter, 1987: 17

Medical superintendents of asylums gradually became psychiatrists, but they did not start out as such. Alongside the dominance of psychiatrists, the concept of mental illness became accepted. In other words, in this account, the profession of psychiatry and its associated technologies of diagnosis and treatment only became possible in the institutional arena opened up by an original act of social rejection.

The Enlightenment was also concerned with an exploration of the individual self. The romantic poets began to explore the imagination and playwrights and novelists began to focus on personality and the inner depths of character, not just on plot. This concern with subjectivity was also seen in philosophy and in the early part of the 20th century gave rise to the disciplines of phenomenology and psychoanalysis

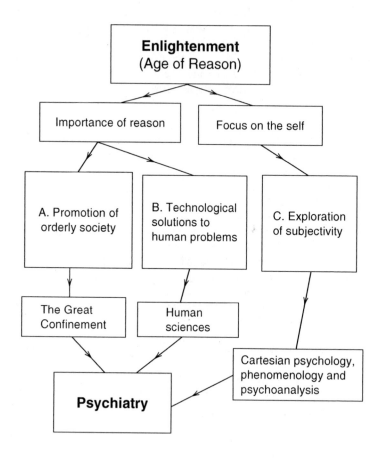

Figure 9.1   The Emergence of Psychiatry from the Age of Reason

In figure 9.1, we have tried to capture the ways in which the cultural transformations of the Age of Reason led directly to the emergence of psychiatry. On the one hand we see the concern with reason leading to confinement, compulsion and coercion in the practical management of people who were deemed to be 'unreasonable'. We also see this concern leading to a belief in science and the technical ordering of our lives and problems. Positivism and the so-called human sciences – psychology, sociology, economics and anthropology – were very much the products of this outlook. They began to replace the religious and aesthetic orientation of the medieval and Renaissance world-view. The doctors who ran the asylums of the 19th century struggled to legitimise their power and prestige by asserting the scientific and medical nature of their theories and treatments. The concern with the interior opened up a territory where 'new discoveries' could be made. Freud, for example, is often portrayed in the guise of an 'explorer of the mind', like Columbus sailing off to chart unknown and dangerous lands in search of new truths. Our argument is that without these cultural developments there would have been no psychiatry.

Twentieth century psychiatry concerned itself with an extension and a refinement of this Enlightenment, or modernist, agenda. Its understanding of distress and madness became even more focused on individuals. It continued to assert a Cartesian understanding of the mind as something separate from the social world around it,[1] and thus separated mental phenomena from background contexts. Psychosis and emotional distress are defined in terms of disordered individual experience. Social and cultural factors are, at best, secondary, and may or may not be taken into account. This is partly because most psychiatric encounters occur in hospitals and clinics, with a therapeutic focus on the individual, with drugs or psychotherapy. It is also because biological, behavioural, cognitive and psychodynamic approaches share a conceptual and therapeutic focus on the individual self.

The technological orientation of psychiatry has also been extended and developed in the 20th century. In many ways the recent 'decade of the brain' epitomises this, based on the assertion that madness is caused by neurological dysfunction that can be cured by drugs targeted at specific neuroreceptors. Simplistic and incredible as this might be, it has now become almost heretical to question this paradigm.

The quest to order distress in a technical idiom can also be seen in the Diagnostic and Statistical Manual (DSM), which defines over 300 mental illnesses, the majority 'identified' in the past 20 years. This has had a powerful effect within psychiatry and psychology but has also extended the influence of this 'technicalisation' of human problems way beyond the traditional boundaries of psychiatric practice. In their book *Making us crazy. DSM: The psychiatric bible and the creation of mental disorders* the American writers, Kutchins & Kirk remark:

> DSM is a guidebook that tells us how we should think about manifestations of sadness and anxiety, sexual activities, alcohol and substance abuse, and many other behaviours. Consequently, the categories created for DSM reorient our thinking about important social matters and affect our social institutions.
>
> Kutchins & Kirk, 1999: 11

When it comes to the third dimension of modernist psychiatry, its coercive nature, we can see how the links between social exclusion, incarceration and psychiatry were forged in the Enlightenment era. In the 20th century, psychiatry's promise to control madness through medical science resonated with the social acceptance of the role of technical expertise. Substantial power was invested in the profession through mental health legislation, which granted psychiatrists the right and responsibility to detain patients and to force them to take powerful drugs, or undergo ECT. Psychopathology and psychiatric nosology became the legitimate framework for these interventions. Despite the enormity of this power, this coercive facet of psychiatry was rarely discussed inside the profession until recently. Psychiatrists are generally keen to downplay the differences between their work and that of their medical colleagues. This emerges in contemporary writing about both stigma and mental health legislation, in which psychiatrists seek to assert the equivalence of psychiatric and medical illness. Ignoring the coercive dimension of psychiatry neither helps the credibility of the discipline nor eases the stigma of mental illness; both patients and public know that, unlike schizophrenia, a diagnosis of diabetes cannot result in them being forced to receive treatment against their wishes.

Challenges to modernist psychiatry

Our position is that a mental health system based on this Enlightenment agenda is no longer tenable. We are confronted with a number of challenges that mean a radical rethinking of our guiding assumptions and orientations is needed.

1   First there are what we call postmodern challenges to the Enlightenment heritage. Postmodern thought does not reject the project of Enlightenment but argues that we need to see its downside as well as its positive aspects. It means questioning simple notions of

progress and advancement and being aware that science can silence as well as liberate.

2 Psychiatry is also challenged by the cultural shift away from modernism. We now live in an era where there is a greater questioning of scientific expertise and authority. This is seen, for example, in the ongoing battle over genetically modified crops and foods. It is also apparent that as a society we are becoming more comfortable with the notion that different perspectives on reality can all have a validity of their own. We are able to live with the idea that there are many different ways of ordering the world, many different paths to the truth and many different ways of thinking about such things as spirituality, health and healing. This is evidenced by the turn to alternative medicine. A recent survey revealed that 20 per cent of GPs in this country practice some form of alternative or complementary medicine.

3 Perhaps of greatest importance is the rise of the user movement over the last 20 years. Users of psychiatry challenge not only the service provision in mental health but they question the theories of psychiatry. While similar to other users of medicine the challenges presented to psychiatry by service users are more fundamental. While patients complain about waiting lists, professional attitudes and poor communication, few would question the enterprise of medicine itself. By contrast, psychiatry has always been thus challenged. Indeed, the concept of mental illness has been described as a myth. It is hard to imagine the emergence of 'anti-paediatrics' or 'critical anaesthetics'; yet anti-psychiatry and critical psychiatry are well-established, influential movements. One of the most influential groups of British mental health service users was called 'Survivors Speak Out'.

4 Government policy has also brought changes to the ethos of mental health care. In Britain, the Labour government has sought (to some extent at least) to tackle links between poverty, unemployment and mental illness which has led to policies that focus on disadvantage and social exclusion.[2] These policies emphasise the importance of contexts, values and partnerships. This is made explicit in the National Service Framework for Mental Health. This raises an agenda that is potentially in conflict with biomedical psychiatry. In a nutshell, the British government (and the society it represents) is asking for a very different kind of psychiatry, and a new deal between professionals and service users.

These developments raise a series of questions which can no longer be ignored:

- If psychiatry is the product of the institution, should we not question its ability to determine the nature of post-institutional care?
- Can we imagine a different relationship between medicine and madness; different, that is, from that forged in the asylums of a previous age?
- If psychiatry is the product of a culture preoccupied with rationality and the individual self, what sort of mental health care is appropriate in the postmodern world in which such preoccupations are waning?
- How appropriate is Western psychiatry for cultural groups who value a spiritual ordering of the world, and an ethical emphasis on the importance of family and community?
- How can we uncouple mental health care from the agenda of social exclusion, coercion and control to which it became bound in the last two centuries?

We believe that if we do not face up to these questions we are in danger of replicating the problems of institutional care in our community services. Indeed, there is evidence that this has already begun to happen with the development of coercive assertive outreach services in Britain and the United States. Relying on the traditional medical approach to understanding madness and distress, these services often see the administration of medication as their most important goal. Other service elements are used to engage users but only in a bid to ensure compliance. As a result, many users have complained that they experience these services as being as oppressive as traditional hospital psychiatry and have begun to campaign against them (Oaks, 1998).

For these reasons, postpsychiatry is driven by a contrasting set of goals.

Postpsychiatry and mental health practice

Postpsychiatry involves a new approach to the mental health practice. It frames the difficulties and challenges we face from a different starting point. Unlike anti-psychiatry and previous forms of critical psychiatry it proposes no new theories about madness. Instead it deconstructs psychiatry and opens up spaces in which alternative understandings of madness can assume the validity denied them by psychiatry. Crucially, it argues that the voices of service users and survivors should be centre stage. This is what we mean by the democratic possibilities of postpsychiatry. In addition, postpsychiatry distances itself from the therapeutic implications of anti-psychiatry. It does not propose new therapies to replace the medical techniques of psychiatry. Anti-psychiatry, especially as developed by R.D. Laing, proposed a modified version of psychoanalysis (based largely on existential philosophy) as an alternative to psychiatry. Others, writing under the heading of 'critical psychiatry', such as Ingleby and Kovel, also looked to different versions of psychoanalysis to frame their theories and practice (Ingleby, 1980b).[3] Postpsychiatry sees the theories of Freud and other analysts as part of the problem, not the solution!

To use a spatial metaphor, postpsychiatry is not a place, a set of fixed ideas and beliefs. Instead, it is more like a set of orientations which together can help us move on from where we are now. It does not to seek to prescribe an end point and does not argue that there are 'right' and 'wrong' ways of tackling madness.

1 Both theoretically and practically postpsychiatry emphasises the importance of *contexts*. We propose that an understanding of the social, political and cultural realities that shape the experiences of those who use mental health services should be primary and central to our understanding of madness and distress. A context-centred approach acknowledges the importance of empirical knowledge in understanding the effects of social factors on individual experience, but it also engages with knowledge from non-Cartesian models of mind, such as those inspired by the philosophers Wittgenstein and Heidegger and the Russian psychologist Vygotsky. We use the term 'hermeneutic' for such knowledge, because priority is given to meaning and interpretation. Events, reactions and social networks are not conceptualised as separate items which can be measured and analysed causally in isolation, but are instead understood as bound together in a web of meaningful connections which can be explored and illuminated, whilst defying simple causal explanation (see, for example, Thomas et al, 2004; Bracken & Thomas, 2005).

2 We also believe that, in practical clinical work, mental health interventions do not have to be based on an individualistic framework centred on medical diagnosis and treatment (Williams et al, 1999; Bracken, 2001). The Hearing Voices Network offers a good example of how very different ways of providing support can be developed. This does not negate the importance of biological or psychological perspectives but it refuses to privilege these and regards them as based on particular assumptions and values, which themselves are derived from a particular context.

3 Postpsychiatry problematises the ever-increasing tendency to medicalise and technicalise our lives and our problems. 'Clinical effectiveness' and 'evidence-based practice'; the idea that science should guide clinical practice, currently dominates medicine. Psychiatry has embraced this agenda in the quest for solutions to its current difficulties. The problem is that clinical effectiveness

downplays the importance of values in research and practice. All medical practice involves a certain amount of negotiation about assumptions and values. However, because psychiatry is primarily concerned with beliefs, moods, relationships and behaviours this negotiation actually constitutes the bulk of its clinical endeavours. Recent work by medical anthropologists and philosophers, has pointed to the values and assumptions which underpin psychiatric classification (Gaines, 1992; Fulford, 1994). Postpsychiatry seeks to put *ethics before technology*. In other words it seeks to expose the ways in which values guide the technologies available in mental health work. If we are aware of these, it becomes possible to debate and discuss them and to see if different values and priorities might be more appropriate. While this is an issue for all mental health work the dangers of ignoring these questions is most apparent in the problematic encounter between psychiatry and non-European populations, both within Europe and elsewhere.

4   Postpsychiatry seeks to *separate issues of care and treatment from the process of coercion*. The extended debate about the new Mental Health Act in Britain has offered an opportunity to rethink the relationship between medicine and madness. Many service users and their organisations question the 'medical model', and are outraged that this provides the framework for coercive care. This is not to say that society should never remove a person's liberty on account of mental disorder. However, by challenging the notion that psychiatric theory is neutral, objective and disinterested, postpsychiatry weakens the case for medical control of the process. Perhaps, doctors should be able to apply for detention (alongside other individuals and groups), but not make the decision to detain someone. In addition, the principle of reciprocity means that legislation must include safeguards such as independent peer advocacy and advance directives.

Democracy, citizenship and postpsychiatry

We have already pointed out that current understandings of madness and distress are dominated by the technological languages of psychiatry and psychology, what Nikolas Rose (1979) has called the 'psy' complex. Our view is that this domination is global and hegemonic (Thomas et al, 2005); it applies no matter what your perspective or how you are situated in society, whether as a user of services, provider, politician, academic or member of the public. In our culture, madness is almost universally discussed in medical terms or in the specialised words of clinical psychology. It is not referred to as a mundane feature of human experience. Those not privy to the specialist languages of the 'psy' complex defer to the expertise of those who have such access. People who experience episodes of madness, alienation and distress are usually told to seek 'professional help'. Consequently there are enormous barriers facing the arguments that we have proposed here, that wider social, cultural and political factors influence and shape our physical and emotional well-being, and that these factors are of prime importance in responding to madness. Housing officers, people working in benefits offices, academics and policy makers defer to the expertise of psychiatrists when it comes to tackling social exclusion.

This is the struggle that groups like Mad Pride and Mad Chicks are engaged in.[4] They argue that much of their suffering arises from society's response to their condition as mad people. There are parallels here with the Gay Rights movement, which early in its history, challenged the idea that homosexuality was an illness. The fight against discrimination, exclusion and oppression took the form of a positive campaign in which gay people struggled to 'define' themselves and develop their own agendas for the future, alongside arguments against the medical framing of homosexuality as some sort of disease was a move to celebrate gay culture.

If groups like Mad Pride are engaged in acts of self-liberation, how does this stand in relation to the actions of governments, policy makers, mental health workers and managers, all of whom are included in this society from which the mad are excluded? In recent years the concept of citizenship has been proposed as a way of challenging social exclusion and moving towards a more inclusive society for those who use mental health services (Sayce, 2000). The medical model postulates that 'diseases' such as schizophrenia lead to social exclusion (unemployment, poor housing and the associated socioeconomic privations) because the disease process prevents the individual from participating effectively in society. This is because of the deterioration in cognitive function thought to be associated with the 'defect state' that is said to be an intrinsic feature of so-called poor prognosis, negative symptom schizophrenia. In other words social exclusion is an outcome of the disease process. Elsewhere we have argued that this is not the case (Thomas, 1997). Adopting a citizenship approach to mental health means that the *reasons* for the relationship between social exclusion and schizophrenia are no longer as important.[5] The fact that such relationships exist at all is the main concern, and this places an obligation on us all to remedy the situation. This is important because it takes the responsibility for tackling social exclusion out of the clinic and into the wider community. As with disabled people and the social model of disability, the situation will only be rectified when society is better organised to enable people who experience psychosis to participate, as full citizens. This means the enactment of anti-discrimination and other legislation to make sure that people who are socially excluded are able to participate fully in society, and are not marginalised or stigmatised.

Marinetto (2003) points out that the idea of citizenship, particularly active citizenship, has re-emerged as a prominent feature of the political discourse of advanced liberal democracies over the last 20 years, and he examines the idea of citizenship critically using Foucault's later work. Foucault coined the term 'governmentality' (1991) to describe a particular type of mentality that characterises state activity in liberal democracies. Its main feature is that the state can, should and must manage and regulate all aspects of society and individual behaviour. This is important in relation to citizenship. The rights we associate with being citizens, such as the right to work, to be housed, to participate in democracy, or to be autonomous self-determining beings, stand in a complex relationship to governmentality. Advanced liberal democracies no longer rely on centralised institutions to foster and maintain the state's power and control over their citizens. This means that to be a citizen is to be free of the centralised authority of the state, but this freedom comes at a price. It means that we are expected to internalise forms of morality and notions of normality, especially in terms of our sexuality and rationality, that is to say in terms of how we are permitted to think and experience the world. Nikolas Rose (1996) sees the government's emphasis on community as part of these regulatory processes. The idea of 'community' has become incorporated into professional and expert discourses and programmes of knowledge. The same can be said of citizenship, which has become a focus for government attempts to deal with complex social and political phenomena like crime, drug misuse immigration and terrorism. As a result a new sector of government has appeared which develops policy programmes which rely on the capabilities of communities. This, according to Rose, is how we may understand active citizenship, where:

> ... new modes of neighbourhood participation, local empowerment and engagement of residents in decisions over their own lives will, it is thought, reactivate self-motivation, self-responsibility and self-reliance.
>
> Rose, 1996: 335, cited in Marinetto, 2003: 109

Seen in this light, citizenship may be seen as a form of government. As Marinetto puts it:

Encouraging active citizenship promotes a particular type of personal morality and positive form of life for communities, individuals and governments.

Marinetto, 2003: 109

Halperin, writing from the perspective of queer politics, puts governmentality this way:

The state no longer needs to frighten or coerce its subjects into proper behaviour: it can safely leave them to make their own choices in the allegedly sacrosanct private sphere of personal freedom which they now inhabit, because within that sphere they *freely and spontaneously* police both their own conduct and the conduct of others – and so 'earn' by demonstrating a capacity to exercise them, the various rights assigned by the state's civil institutions exclusively to law-abiding citizens possessed of sound minds and bodies.

Halperin, 1995: 18-19

In this sense we can see active citizenship as a governmental strategy for regulating the population, which, by virtue of the fact that it appears not to be centralised, conveys the impression of decentred government.[6] This is important in understanding the relationship between citizenship and madness. Halperin's caveat, that the rights assigned by the state are granted '... exclusively to law-abiding citizens possessed of sound minds and bodies' suggests that citizenship in relation to madness remains conditional. It remains tied to a particular view of reality, one that excludes madness. The prevailing moral order privileges those subjectivities that are essentially Cartesian and rationalist. Any other form of subjectivity is excluded and relegated to the hinterlands that are patrolled and policed by psychology and psychiatry. Thus a Foucauldian analysis of power and governmentality suggests that citizenship in advanced liberal democracies is tightly bound up with hegemonic judgements about what is and what is not rational. As long as citizenship remains tied to particular 'normalised' conceptions of rational subjectivity (for example that the experience of hearing voices is only to be understood as a symptom of schizophrenia) then its ability to overcome the social exclusion experienced by the mad will be limited. Citizenship should be inclusive; people should not be excluded simply because they do not experience reality in the way that the majority do.

So, the question raised here concerns the type of values, morality and 'positive form(s) of life' (to quote Marinetto) promoted by active citizenship and the 'decentred' government. It may appear that there is no longer an authoritative state telling us how to lead our lives, or how we should interpret and makes sense of our lives and our relationships, but it seems to us that the forces of governmentality that shape our subjectivities are becoming increasingly diffuse and ambiguous. The notion of the monolithic centralised state which dictated political, cultural, aesthetic and moral norms to its citizens, as happened under Stalinism in the former Soviet Union, has passed into history. Instead we have something less tangible. Indeed the various processes associated with globalisation – the growth of transnational capitalism and the market, mass migration, the increasingly porous boundaries between cultures – all these factors have shattered the idea of the self-contained nation state. Increasingly we are forced to position ourselves on one side or another of conflicts that out-strip national boundaries. 'You are either with us or against us', either against terrorism, or if not, we are seen as standing in opposition to 'freedom' and 'democracy', or more cynically, the global interests of the US economy dominated by the twin towers of the arms and pharmaceutical industry. The global pharmaceutical industry is flooding the world with the view that we should interpret ourselves not as sad or demoralised, but as depressed. This is one example of how are we encouraged to think about ourselves in ways that are not necessarily in our best interests.

Conclusion

In the past psychiatry reacted defensively to challenges and, throughout the 20th century, has asserted its medical identity. However, while the discipline survived the anti-psychiatry of the 1960s, as we have seen, fundamental questions about its legitimacy remain. The so-called 'failure' of community care and the British government's response (in the form of the National Service Framework, and proposed changes to the mental health act) make it essential that we critically re-examine psychiatric frameworks. Psychiatry, like medicine, will have to adapt to the 'postmodern environment' in which we now live and to the reality of the user movement. This is not going to go away. Twenty years ago homosexuality was still defined as a disease by the Diagnostic and Statistical Manual (DSM) in the US. The movement for gay rights was small and easily dismissed. The idea that in the future there would be TV programmes made for gay people by gay people or that a number of cabinet ministers would be openly gay would have been dismissed as laughable. We don't know at this stage how the user movement will develop, but develop and expand it will.

Postpsychiatry seeks to 'democratise' the field of mental health by linking progressive service development to a debate about contexts, values and partnerships. The advent of postmodernity offers an exciting challenge for doctors and other professionals involved in this area and represents an opportunity to rethink our roles and responsibilities. We look forward to a situation where experiences such as hearing voices, depression, fearfulness, withdrawal and self-harm are no longer conceptualised as purely medical issues. Contrary to the prevailing approach within psychiatry we believe that we will reduce the stigma of madness and distress only by demedicalising the field. However, giving up the frameworks and models we have become used to is not without its difficulties. Framing our lives and distress in a medical way has its immediate advantages. But then the struggle for democracy has never been easy. We believe that traditional psychiatry has served to narrow our focus. It has limited our imagination and restricted our vision of how we as individuals and communities can care for one another in times of distress and dislocation, withdrawal and despair. Increasingly it binds us to the powerful agenda of global capitalism. We need something different. We need an agenda that is thoughtful, critical and democratic.

Notes

1   A more detailed account of these aspects of psychiatry can be found in Bracken & Thomas (2005), particularly chapters four and five.
2   See for example the report: *Mental Health and Social Exclusion* published by the Social Exclusion Unit in 2004.
3   See Thomas & Bracken (2004) for a more detailed comparison of anti-psychiatry, critical psychiatry and postpsychiatry.
4   See www.madpride.org.uk/
5   This is an example of what we mean by prioritising ethics over technology. Positivism, or the application of science (in this case in psychiatry) to the human experience of psychosis, results in the generation of categories such as schizophrenia. Scientific logic demands that questions of causality are of prime importance, and for this reason psychiatric knowledge is concerned to explain the link between negative symptoms and 'social deterioration'. In postpsychiatry ethical questions about the relationship are prioritised, such as what are the most appropriate ways of remedying such situations
6   Marinetto, though, questions whether this is actually the case. He points out that central government, and other public authorities have

immense power and control, through writing policies and gate-keeping resources that control and influence citizenship and community participation.

10

The Biopsychological Approach in Psychiatry: The Meyerian Legacy

D.B. Double

When giving notice of a memorial service for the eminent psychiatrist Theodore Lidz, the *Yale Bulletin and Calendar* (2001) observed that Lidz had expressed regret in his last years that he did not write just one more book to show that biology-based lines of research and training in current psychiatry are 'barking up the wrong tree'. Lidz was professor and chief of clinical services in psychiatry at Yale, having taken his residency in psychiatry at Johns Hopkins University, where he studied with Adolf Meyer. There is no question about his distinguished standing within mainstream psychiatry. Although he was critical of the biomedical model of mental illness, this did not mean that his views were labelled and dismissed as 'anti-psychiatry'.

Lidz's perspective in psychiatry, based in the Meyerian tradition, emphasised continuities between normal development and psycho-pathology. He saw it as essential to focus on the individual's life history to understand patients in the context of familial, community and cultural factors that affect personality development. He appreciated the extent to which mental illness is induced by early experience in troubled families. This biopsychological approach was developed before the emergence of anti-psychiatry.

Despite Lidz's orthodoxy, the affinity between his position and anti-psychiatry was recognised by Boyers & Orrill (1972) when they chose to interview him for their edited collection of what they considered at the time to be most of the serious writing that had been addressed to the work of R.D. Laing. In the interview, Lidz identified various excesses in the work of Laing, but he made clear that he did not consider schizophrenia to be an organic disease and instead viewed it as a developmental reaction related to personality organisation.

Like Laing, Lidz had been involved in family studies of schizophrenic patients. Lidz viewed schizophrenia as an extreme form of social withdrawal, specifically characterised by efforts to modify reality into a tenable form by distorting symbolisation of reality, or through extreme limitation of the interpersonal environment (Lidz et al, 1957). Data was collected from schizophrenic families over several years using multiple methods involving weekly interviews with family members; observation of interaction with each other and staff; projective testing and other techniques. All families were found to communicate defectively. The essence of the problem was thought to be the egocentricity of the dominant parent or sometimes both parents that prevented the parent from understanding and treating the child as a separate and discrete individual, rather than as part of the parent or as someone whose essential function is to complete a parent's life or salvage the parents' marriage. There was either a schismatic conflict in the parents' marriage that divided the family into two camps and that resulted in each spouse destroying the worth of the other; or the family was seen as distorted by a skew in the marital relationship by the passive acceptance of the serious psychopathology of the dominant spouse by the other, with masking of the serious problems that arise, creating an aberrant environment that confuses the child.

Lidz (1972) complained that when Laing discussed mystification in the family that he did not make reference to his and his colleagues' work that covered similar ground dealing with irrational patterns of communication in the family. As far as Lidz was concerned, the work by Singer & Wynne (1965) on communication problems in the family was more influential than Laing's contribution. Lidz pointed out that Adolf Meyer had advocated taking experience as a fact in itself, which is close to Laing's perspective and that very little of what Laing proposed was new.

What I want to do in this chapter is to discuss the biopsychological approach in relation to the biomedical perspective. Like Lidz, I want to suggest that Laing and so-called 'anti-psychiatry' were not really providing a new perspective. There were some excesses in anti-psychiatry (see chapter 2), but the biopsychological approach has a long history, even if it has only ever been a minority viewpoint within psychiatry. I will look at the historical origins of this interpretative perspective and discuss the work of Adolf Meyer and its relation to anti-psychiatry.

Historical origins

This historical narrative is necessarily selective and schematic. It is more of a genealogy, attempting to make theories about the concept of mental illness intelligible. However, it does set a context for the understanding of the origins of biomedical and biopsychological perspectives. It is necessary to go into reasonable detail to appreciate these foundations.

Many different views of the origins of mental illness have been promulgated in history. For example, in the 18th century, disturbances of blood and its circulation were frequently cited as causes of mania and melancholia. Friedreich Hoffmann, for instance, attributed both these diseases to insufficient perfusion of the brain, the extent of which determined whether it was mania or melancholia that occurred. Similarly, Benjamin Rush, often regarded as the father of American psychiatry, thought that the cause of madness 'is seated primarily in the blood-vessels of the brain, and depends upon the same kind of morbid and irregular actions that constitute other arterial diseases' (Rush, 1962).

Our modern views of mental illness can probably best be dated to 1845 when both Griesinger's *Die Pathogie und Therapie der psychischen Krankheiten* and Feuchtersleben's *Lehrbuch der ärztlichen Seelenkunde* were published. Griesinger is commonly seen as the primary representative of biomedical psychiatry. Similarly, I want to suggest that Feuchtersleben should be seen as the originator of the biopsychological perspective. These authors took the mind–body debate forward from the somaticist–mentalist conflict that had been in contention in psychiatry for several decades. To put their views in context, we need to have some appreciation of this historical debate.

The mentalists' position was exemplified by J.C. Heinroth's statement that 'in psychical disorders, the soul is directly taken ill, and the origins of this illness lie in sin; the physical suffering involved is more of a coincidental and secondary nature'. From this perspective, mind was separated from brain, and in particular the philosophical and medical concept of mind was conflated with the theological concept of soul in a way that was more Cartesian than our modern understanding. It no longer makes sense from our modern world-view to suggest that sin is the cause of mental illness. What happened with Griesinger and Feuchtersleben was that it became manifest that the soul was no longer relevant to the description of mental illness.

For the somaticists, of which Johannes Baptista Friedreich was a staunch supporter (Kirkby, 1992), the soul as such could not 'directly become diseased'. Friedreich viewed the soul predominantly in the ideal, metaphysical sense as immutable and immortal and therefore, as far as he was concerned, it did not make sense to regard it as diseased. Instead, a lesion in a somatic organ was seen as the root cause of psychic disease, generally via its effect on the brain. All somatic diseases, including diseases of the brain and nervous system, could lead to the development of psychic disease. Psychic affectations, such as the passions or affects, only cause psychic disease through a somatic intermediary, for example anxiety and sadness predominantly influence the heart and liver, and so forth.

Wilhelm Griesinger's followers were the successors to the somaticists, but there was an important difference. The former believed that intra-cerebral factors were important. The latter held that the cause of mental disorders lay in other bodily organs (Beer, 1996). In other words, Griesinger went a stage further and adopted an explicitly materialistic position. To quote from him: 'It is only from a neuropathological standpoint that one can try to make sense of the symptomatology of the insane.' Disturbances of the soul or mind were no longer seen as secondary to another process, but rather as manifestations of a neuropathological entity. This is essentially the same principle as our modern biomedical perspective.

Griesinger's statement, which became a slogan, that 'mental diseases are diseases of the brain', did not in fact imply that all psychopathology was an expression of neuroanatomical changes (Marx, 1972). He was not as thoroughgoing in his reductionism as may commonly be assumed. For Griesinger, mental illness in its initial phase was characterised by psychopathology that was not accompanied by structural brain changes and hence was reversible. Mental factors were, therefore, seen to be of primary importance in causing mental illness and this functional concept did not pose a theoretical problem for his model. Structural changes only occurred in what he called the second phase, in which mental image formation or will was affected, and also in the third phase, which implied deterioration and incurability.

Ernst von Feuchtersleben (1976) praised Griesinger's book but questioned whether 'mental disorders were always due only to disorders of the brain'. Feuchtersleben simplified the whole issue of psyche and soma and their interdependence by claiming mind as the meeting place of body and spirit (Burns, 1954). He saw mental illness as a functional disorder, and, in this sense, mind has 'no seat' (Laor, 1982). He regarded metaphysical questions, such as whether or not the spirit can become diseased, as inconsequential. It is important not to misunderstand this position. Feuchtersleben was not suggesting that mental illness is a mere metaphor, as was suggested by Szasz (1972), but instead that it is a psychophysical functional disturbance, which of course has a biological basis.

It was Feuchtersleben who coined the term 'psychosis' to denote 'mental disorder which affected the personality as a whole' (Beer, 1995). Carl Fuerstner later employed the term 'functional psychosis' in 1881 for mental disorders without somatic signs, contrasting these psychoses with general paralysis, and again made no attempt to make psychosis a materialistic notion. In its origin, then, 'psychosis' is a biopsychological concept.

In the course of the 19th century, evidence for anatomical pathology accumulated in clinical cases of insanity, albeit in a minority. Both Griesinger and Feuchtersleben were writing not long before Virchow's *Cellular pathology* in 1858 initiated a new era in medicine and medical research (Marx, 1972). Virchow's focus on the individual elements of cells created a foundation in histology for modern pathology. As more was discovered about the workings of the brain, there seemed to be less room for any contribution from a Cartesian soul, which became redundant. Increasingly a psychophysical parallelism was championed, in which mental processes and symptoms were the secondary and epiphenomenal signs of bodily process or disease.

By 1897, Alois Alzheimer could state that evidence of physical abnormalities was unequivocal in dementia paralytica, senile dementia, the various focal diseases of the brain, imbecility and idiocy. With the discovery in 1905 of *Treponema pallidum* in the inguinal glands of patients with dementia paresis and the subsequent introduction of the Wasserman test, he was able to firm up his category of organic psychosis, meaning those disorders with positive histological findings. He later added Kraepelin's new disease of dementia praecox (which was renamed schizophrenia by Eugene Bleuler) to the organic conditions, although manic-depressive insanity was listed as functional.

Alzheimer himself was critical of more thoroughgoing biomedical views such as those of Franz Nissl, who rejected the juxtaposition of the organic and functional psychoses and regarded all psychoses of whatever type as always having positive cortical findings. Nonetheless many late 19th-century psychiatrists and neurologists used the term 'functional' to denote conditions that although they had no gross anatomical changes were nevertheless thought to have 'sub-anatomical', molecular disturbances.

This perspective set the trend for 20th-century assumptions about the biomedical basis of psychosis. By the later editions of *General psychopathology*, Jaspers (1963) reserved the term psychosis for definite disease processes. The functional psychoses of genuine epilepsy, schizophrenia and manic-depressive illness were identified by their lack of organic findings. Schneider (1959) preferred the term endogenous to functional psychosis, making clear that he assumed an undiscovered organic aetiology for endogenous psychosis. This hypothesis still underlies modern biomedical views.

Alongside these biomedical developments, biopsychological influences were also at work, although these trends perhaps always represented a minority view. Grob (1963) contrasts the materialism of the latter half of the 19th century, which emphasised structural pathology producing a therapeutic pessimism, with the progressive outlook at the end of the 19th century and early 20th century, characterised by an optimistic moralism and a belief that the individual could be changed by altering his/her social environment. In this context, Adolf Meyer (1866-1950), an immigrant to the United States from Switzerland, offered a new view of mental disorders, distinct both from the nosological views of Emil Kraepelin and the psychoanalytic movement developed from Sigmund Freud. Building on the philosophical approaches of Charles S. Pierce, William James and John Dewey, Meyer developed a dynamic psychology based on the pragmatic method, which James (1907) called 'primarily a method of settling metaphysical disputes that otherwise might be interminable'. In other words, Meyer sought an integration of mind and brain that avoided this philosophical dilemma.

The development of psychoanalysis from Sigmund Freud reinforced the notion that mental symptoms may have meaning by making explicit its view about the psychogenic origins of functional illness. Furthermore, human elements were still influential despite institutional pressures in the asylums. Efforts to make the treatment of the insane more humane, such as those of Dorothea Lynde Dix and other reformers, challenged the abuses of restraint and isolation. The mental hygiene movement, initiated by the experiences of treatment in confinement by Clifford Beers (1908), aimed to improve understanding of the mental patient. As the numbers of people in the asylums continued to increase, the creation of an atmosphere of a therapeutic community became identified as an important element in treatment (World Health Organisation, 1953), heralding the opening of the locked doors in mental hospitals.

These trends focusing on the person counterbalanced the biomedical perspective and provided the sources for the biopsychological approach, which I want to consider in more detail. In particular, the work of Adolf Meyer, which was called psychobiology, is central to this development.

Psychobiology

Before discussing the concepts of psychobiology, a word of warning is required about Adolf Meyer's style of communication in English. Although he lived in the United States for many years, the expression of his ideas could be convoluted and tortuous. I am not exactly sure of the reason for this. I have consulted his collected papers in The Alan Mason

Chesney Medical Archives of the Johns Hopkins Medical Institutions (Leys, 1999). Some of his correspondence is relatively well written and I am not sure whether his secretary corrected the English after dictation. His published writings are not always as easy to follow as some of these letters. I came across a heartfelt note written in the early hours of the morning towards the end of his life (November 1947).

> Wherein did I fail? Did I?
> What is the problem?
> With whom? How? in-between and all the prepositions that suggest themselves and arise or can be raised and applied – personal self or other, through – by – because of – etc
>
> Meyer Archives Series VI/8/199

This note may be seen as Meyer's appreciation of his own communication difficulties. He struggled for years to get his 1932 Salmon Memorial lectures into print and the task required considerable editorial assistance, leading to the adapted lectures eventually being published posthumously (Meyer, 1957). Otherwise he wrote no books; his writings in journals, many of them originally given as lectures for specific purposes, were eventually collected and published in four volumes (Winters, 1950, 1951). Meyer himself recognised his failure to be explicit about his psychiatric system. I will return to this issue in the conclusion when discussing the oppositional nature of anti-psychiatry in comparison to the more harmonious, compromising position of Meyer. At this stage, however, I merely want to prepare the reader for some difficult passages in some of the quotations from Meyer, which I think are necessary to appreciate his writings fully.

Psychobiology was a term introduced by Adolf Meyer for the study of man as a person within the framework of biology (Muncie, 1939). As Meyer said, 'The object of our study is, literally, an indivisible individual' (Meyer, 1957). The traditional medical student in his/her first days of medical school was confronted with a body for dissection. The focus of training was on the dysfunction of more or less detachable bodily parts and organs. Instead, psychobiology concentrates on the reactions of a unitary organism, mentally integrated through symbolisation and consciousness. Symbolisation is the process by which time-bound experience is meaningfully represented, creating the capacity for influencing present and future experience. Consciousness is the awareness of personal activities, and is a matter of degree rather than absolutely separate from 'not-conscious'. In many ways, Meyer anticipates the more recent emphasis on patient-centred medicine (Stewart et al, 2003).

Adolf Meyer's chief quest was for a better solution to the mind–body problem – ie. a functional understanding of this interaction. The theoretical basis of his philosophy was pragmatism and pluralism. These particularly American contributions to the history of thought provided a stimulus to develop his biopsychological approach. In his own words:

> William James' clear vision of the significance of the 'pragmatism' of Charles S. Pierce and the 'instrumentalism' of John Dewey, and the healthy encouragement given to natural spontaneity of thought and work in the American environment, were all sympathetic to a realignment of concepts in harmony with what was essentially an urge to place one's confidence in the potency of experience.
>
> Meyer, 1957: 47

Meyer, therefore, created an overarching holistic, unitary personality theory. He avoided the dangers of reductionism, by refusing to reduce mental events to physical activity. On the other hand, he also avoided degeneration into relativism by proposing that his commonsense approach amounted to an organised body of facts, methods of study and methods of therapeutic procedure. His integrative vision was that:

> We do not have to be mind-shy or body-shy any longer. Today we can attack the facts as we find them, without that disturbing obsession of having to translate them first into something artificial before we can study them and work with them. Since we have reached a sane pluralism with a justifiable conviction of the fundamental consistency of it all, a satisfaction with what we modestly call formulation rather than definition and with an appreciation of relativity, we have at last an orderly and natural field and method from which nobody need shy.

It is important to realise that Meyer was not excluding biological factors. He trained as a neurologist. He was well aware of the role that the brain plays in behavioural disorders. A way to make clear his appreciation of the influence of the brain in functional mental disorder is to quote from a 1942 post-retirement note in his archives: 'All person disorders must show *through* the brain but not always *in* the brain [his emphasis]' (Meyer Archives Series I/3051/1). In other words, Meyer was dissatisfied with a parallelism of mind and body. He recognised the potency of mental processes and did not regard them as mere epiphenomena. Nonetheless he was clear about the biological mediation of mental disorders through the brain.

Meyer emphasised the need for what he called a 'critical common sense'. By this he meant:

a preference for what can be observed by any competent person, with freedom from mere dogmaticism and dictation and domination.

There are echoes in this notion of more modern understandings, such as the need to promote critical thinking and reflective practice in medicine (Maudsley & Strivens, 2000; Mamede & Schmidt, 2004).

By 'critical common sense' Meyer also meant a 'frankly functional consideration' of the concreteness of the patient's story. This emphasis, again, predates more modern trends with the same focus, such as narrative based medicine (Greenhalgh & Hurwitz, 1998). The central element is the presentation of the narrative 'as data of observation within a responsible experiment'. In Meyer's own words, again:

The strongest influence in my own work was the sensing of the importance and need for a psychology based on practical demands, an interpretative understanding rather than an abstract psychology and psychiatry disregarding function by meaning. Even at the turn of the century in Worcester I had been interested in the story, and I saw no virtue in making an academic distinction which left content and meaning solely to the novelist

Meyer, 1957: 45

Meyer's broad emphasis meant that he did not restrict his outlook to what was happening in the asylums. His interest in the origins of mental disorder created a focus on mental health promotion, which he built on the development of public hygiene and for which he coined the term 'mental hygiene'. The mental hygiene movement had its inception in the experiences of Clifford Beers (1908), who approached Meyer for support to improve conditions in asylums, based on his own adverse experiences of his treatment for his manic-depressive illness. The US National Committee for Mental Hygiene was formed in 1909 and the first International Congress on Mental Hygiene was held in 1930.

Meyer had a clear appreciation of the social aspects of psychiatry. He met the people of Hull-House, the most influential social settlement house in America. His wife developed an interest in volunteer service, visiting patients' homes and speaking to their relatives – the first psychiatric social worker. 'I was greatly assisted by the wholesome human understanding of my helpmate.' She gave him an awareness of the situation to which a patient would return upon discharge. 'In a short time her work became absolutely indispensable.' Mrs. Meyer then channelled her sympathetic intelligence into occupational therapy. She introduced work into the wards as a systematic activity and also organised recreation and encouraged patients in folk dancing as a form of group therapy.

There are several implications of the principles resulting from Meyer's focus on the centrality of the person. They cover at least three areas and I want to consider these in turn: (1) scientific method; (2) the role of psychiatric diagnosis; and (3) the relation between psychoanalysis and psychobiology.

Scientific method

For Meyer, scientific study should include all those functions that are distinctively and uniquely human. Mechanistic psychologies, such as introspection-associationist and behaviourist-conditioned reflex approaches, are not based on an adequate and logically tenable philosophy. This is because of their exclusion of personal factors.

Meyer appointed John B. Watson, the celebrated behaviourist, to his department to teach psychology on the medical course. This shows Meyer's open-minded approach, allowing Watson to push his behaviourist theory to its limits. However, Meyer was clear that Watson's efforts were doomed to failure, at least in the area of psychopathology. This is evidenced by correspondence between them in 1916 (Meyer Archives Series I/3974/9-11). Meyer saw Watson's attempt to exclude every reference to the mental or the psyche as nonsensical. His initial reaction to a paper by Watson on 'What is mental disease?' was expressed in an unreserved way in a draft letter to Watson, but perhaps typically was never sent as such:

> Your application of the concept of conditioned reflexes is acceptable enough as far as it attempts to make fairly clear what the term may be made to mean; but to use it as a formulation with the character of a dogma of exclusive salvation is a mere evasion of a psychophobic nature ... I consider the attitude immature and suspect it of being hopelessly narrow, another one of those panaceas which make an impression on some students and create confusion in a good many more.

More generally, Meyer set out his understanding of science as shown in figure 10.1. There is a certain hierarchical relation of the various disciplines, with the lower or simpler categories being pertinent to, but not explanatory for, higher or more complex categories. For example, chemistry and physics are relevant to biology, but perhaps with rare exceptions the 'lower' sciences do not provide an adequate explanation for biological phenomena, which require a new sort of explanation.

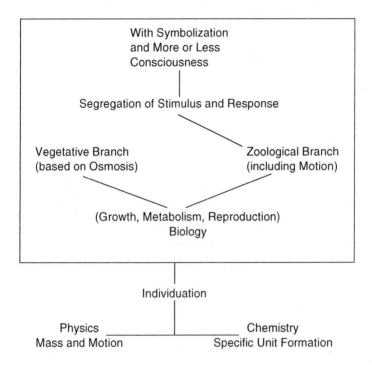

Figure 10.1 Meyer's Understanding of Science

The different scientific disciplines are relatively discontinuous because of qualitative differences in their subject matter and limitations in the methods of study. Individuation first appears in biology beyond physics and chemistry. Within biology are the subdivisions of botany and zoology. Human beings emerge as a special and a higher biological product. Psychobiology demands knowledge of the physical sciences and of anatomy and physiology, but these in no way fully explain the phenomena under investigation.

The incorporation of personal material into scientific methods and procedures raises the question as to whether 'the psychobiological approach' can still validly be regarded as science. To quote from Meyer, 'the answer to this question is, to my mind, a matter of relativities and not of finalities' (Meyer, 1957). As far as he was concerned, psychobiology respects the principle of science by observing 'the facts as they are and as they work in and for the life of the person', even if psychobiology is not a science in the natural scientific sense. In essence, Meyer took over the Huxleyan notion of science as being organised commonsense. Research is therefore a general concept – the work required to clear up open questions, rather than only that which can be established through empirical experimentation. Meyer was not a positivist and hoped that science would no longer be restricted to a physical basis. His view was that it was 'unfortunate that science still adheres to an effete and impossible contrast between mental and physical'.

In his teaching, Meyer encouraged students to undertake a thoroughgoing investigation of a single personality, usually themselves. Psychology was incorporated into the medical curriculum in this idiographic way and the course was begun at John Hopkins Medical School in 1913-14 (Meyer 1912). The life chart was introduced as a graphic summary of the events in the person's life, placed alongside a scale of calendar years from birth. Resistance by students to self-searching was recognised and expected. The 'commonsense' nature of the material produced and the emphasis on personal narrative are indicative of Meyer's methods.

The role of psychiatric diagnosis

Meyer (1896) reviewed the fifth edition of Emil Kraepelin's textbook on psychiatry. Even then Meyer found several assertions 'decidedly dogmatic at first sight'. As is well known, Kraepelin went on to delimit two major groups of psychiatric disorders – manic-depressive illness and dementia praecox – through his method of studying the longitudinal outcome of patients. This aid to classification was, and still is, regarded as a major advance in psychiatry. Meyer on the other hand was more cautious. Although he praised Kraepelin's clinical skills, he emphasised that Kraepelin's categories did not exhaust the different presentations and were best viewed as paradigms. 'We should discriminate what can be definitely identified as manic-depressive insanity, or as dementia praecox, but not extend the scope of these terms to merely set up a new kind of arbitrary confusion.'

Moreover, Meyer objected to Kraepelin's assertion that it was time to create disease entities in psychiatry. Already, in the review of the fifth edition of Kraepelin's textbook, Meyer (1906) criticised the arbitrariness of calling dementia praecox a disorder of metabolism. Instead of proposing a disease process, Meyer suggested that every individual is capable of reacting to a very great variety of situations in the social environment by a limited number of reaction types. He developed the notion of habit formation, which becomes progressively self-defeating in mental disorders, motivated by some form of escape, such as daydreaming as a substitute for reality.

Kraepelin's view of dementia praecox as a disease entity created a pessimistic assessment of prognosis. This was countered by Meyer's emphasis on process, implying that deviations of function could be reversed. Kraepelin (1921) did eventually come to accept that his dementia praecox category did not inevitably imply deterioration of the personality. This change of definition had an effect on diagnostic patterns in Kraepelin's Heildelberg clinic, reducing the number of admissions diagnosed as dementia praecox to 18 per cent from a peak of 51 per cent.

Meyer's opinion of Kraepelin is apparent in correspondence he had with Ernst Jones in 1911 (Meyer Archives I/1962/3). Jones made fun of Kraepelin's insistence on the vital importance of the distinction between dementia praecox and manic-depressive illness, yet having broken down practically all the distinctions between them.

> At the last meeting of the Deutsche Verein, at Stuttgart, he [Kraepelin] made the following admission from his unconscious: 'I suppose the Freudians would say the reason why I do not accept their views is that I am suffering from auto-erotic Grossenwahn'. Whether they said it before or not, they will certainly say it now, for it is impolite to contradict such a great authority.

Meyer replied that 'the little utterance of his will greatly amuse Mrs Meyer, and ... coincides too well with her own estimate of the man gained on a Sunday afternoon visit to his country place.' Meyer eventually managed to emancipate himself from 'what residuals of German psychiatry still cling to me', so that Kraepelinian nosology was hardly any longer discussed in his teaching.

Meyer emphasised the psychogenic explanation of mental disorders, trying to understand the reasons for human action. 'We do not think of disease entities but of processes, that is, miscarriages and deviations of functions.' Traditional psychiatric diagnosis, therefore, will inevitably fall short of an appreciation of the aetiology of mental disorder in personal and social contexts. 'Psychiatry has not reached and probably never will reach, the stage where a small number of one-word diagnoses would be more than a formal index.' As a consequence, Meyer was not primarily interested in coming to a formal psychiatric diagnosis when evaluating patients. He has thus been accused of devaluing the whole process of psychiatric diagnosis. His answer to this charge would have been that overvaluing psychiatric diagnosis creates unrealistic expectations of what can be achieved in terms of aetiology and prognosis. It is wrong to feel 'satisfied with the conviction of quiz medicine'.

In summary:

> The following questions must therefore be answered: 'What is the faulty reaction? What are the conditions that led to it? How does it react to special tests and attempts at modification? What can we expect to achieve, and what are the steps to be taken?'

Meyer was more thoroughgoing in his psychodynamic understanding than Eugene Bleuler (1951) who coined the term schizophrenia, which replaced Kraepelin's notion of dementia praecox. Bleuler was the successor to Forel, Meyer's mentor, at the Burghozli Clinic in Switzerland, and came to the conclusion that dementia praecox was an organic disease whose secondary (mental) symptoms were explained by psychoanalytic mechanisms. Here Meyer differed, and he made no distinction between neurotic and psychotic disorders in the sense that all mental disorders should be understood in terms of their psychological origins, even if psychosis may be more difficult to understand in context than neurosis.

Meyer introduced the term 'ergasiology', an ugly term, from the Greek *ergon* meaning energy. He thought there was a need to create new terminology because the word 'behaviour' has no plural or satisfactory adjective and is apt to exclude cognitive aspects. 'Ergasias are the behavioristically conceived overt and implicit products of psychobiological integration, the human factors taken for granted by common sense when we speak of the actions, reactions and attitudes of the "he" or "she" ' (Meyer, 1957).

He created a classificatory system of particular kinds of reaction types, denoted by terms sharing the suffix 'ergasia'. For example, thymergasias were the affective disorders, and parergasias were schizophrenia and paranoid states. This made the scheme unnecessarily difficult to understand and it never became generally accepted. However, the first edition of the American Diagnostic and Statistical Manual (DSM-I) was influenced by Meyer's notion of reaction types, even if the scheme did not fully accept his terminology.

The relation between psychoanalysis and psychobiology

Like psychoanalysis, Meyer had a dynamic psychological understanding. Both psychobiology and psychoanalysis have a respect for context. Both accept that meaning does make a difference and is variously operative.

The events of mental life are an important realm of functioning. The subject is differentiated through the function of signs. Verbal reports on subjective states are indicators of mental processes. There is agreement between psychoanalysis and psychobiology on these points.

Although Meyer had no objection to working with Freudian concepts, he preferred the freedom of using the trained critical commonsense that he valued. He objected to Freudian determinism, because as far as he was concerned chance and accident evidently do exist. Meyer had a much more relative understanding of concepts than the all-or-none principles of psychoanalysis. For Meyer, it is important not to disregard the essential psychobiological facts of a case, and the continual search for what was latent behind the manifest content reminded Meyer of 'the kind of quest for the Platonic reality'. He was critical of the mystical character of psychoanalytic technique and called psychoanalysis a cult with its promise of salvation. For Meyer, the overemphasis on sex symbolism was incorrect. In summary, in his own words:

I consider psychoanalysis a most noteworthy and highly fruitful venture in the development of medicine, with generalizations made fascinating through the utilization of one particular type of human relation, that of sexual love. But with all my appreciation for a master-creation of the art of dramatization and analogy, psychiatric experience shows that it is by no means so exclusive a way to salvation as the popularizing statements would seem to claim. And with all my respect for the domain which has been characterized as 'the unconscious', and thus relatively inaccessible except through specially devised methods and techniques, I prefer to urge the common sense psychobiological approach which starts from what is accessible and views symptoms as a real part of an attempt at adjustment.

Freud first spoke publicly on psychoanalysis in the USA at Clark University in 1909 (Freud, 1910). At the same convocation, Meyer (1910) delivered his lecture 'The dynamic interpretation of dementia praecox', to which Freud and Jung listened 'in a very absent-minded way' (Meyer Archives VI/8/201). Freud always regarded the American influence on psychoanalysis as superficial, diluting its orthodoxy. Meyer saw the development of dynamic psychology quite differently and challenged Freud's interpretation.

Objections to psychobiology

In manner, Meyer was unassuming, dignified and courteous (Gelder, 1991). He could be intimidating, and his energy and enthusiasm meant he was in charge until his early 70s at the Phipps Clinic, where he was the first director from when it opened at the Johns Hopkins hospital in 1913. His mission in psychiatry was very influential in America, and came to Britain via Aubrey Lewis and David Henderson (Gelder, 1991). Yet his inspiration had faded at the Phipps Clinic a few years after his death when visited by Michael Shepherd (1986).

Even in life, Meyer may not have always had the authority for his views as may be assumed. For example, an article written by John C. Whitehorn in 1936 sent in correspondence to Meyer suggested that 'some of the most influential leaders of the national psychiatric society tried to dissuade Meyer from presenting his views in their meetings on the ground that his maudlin remarks [about Kraepelin] were not scientific psychiatry'. Meyer wrote to Whitehorn thanking him for including his paper: 'I had not known I had created those appearances ... My interest is certainly the scientific material and not the saving of my reputation' (Meyer Archives I/4026/6).

Few references are now made to Meyer's writings in the literature. Although Meyer's ideas never really took hold as a systematic theory of psychiatry (O'Neill, 1980), under his influence American psychiatry came to have a distinctively pragmatic, instrumental and pluralistic approach. For example, in the immediate post-war years, Karl Menninger's (1963) *The Vital Balance* represented a broadly conceived psychosocial theory of psychopathology. Menninger regarded Meyer's efforts, together with those of William Alanson White (1933), superintendent of the Government Hospital for the Insane in Washington and Professor of Psychiatry of George Washington University and a man known for his eloquence, as influential forces in producing a unitary concept of mental illness.

What has happened to this pluralistic consensus? The modern perception of Meyer tends to be disparaging and follows the conclusion of Slater & Roth (1969): 'heuristically the Meyerian approach was almost entirely sterile'. Since the 1970s biomedical psychiatry has reasserted its dominance over psychoanalysis and the Meyerian approach (Double, 2005b). In retrospect, the view that mental illnesses have primarily psychological causes could be regarded as a brief interlude (between about 1900 and 1970) in the history of psychiatry (Roth & Kroll, 1986).

Psychobiology was challenged even in its heyday. Muncie (1939) discusses some of the main arguments at the time and I think it is worth revisiting these issues to appreciate the way in which psychobiology could be undermined. I also summarise the defence of psychobiology from Muncie (1939) to these objections.

1 *In refusing to accept the Kraepelinian conceptions, psychobiology has traded Kraepelinian clarity for unclear muddy ideas.*
  Kraepelinian clarity is achieved at the expense of the facts. Any systematisation must include dynamic understanding rather than avoid it.

2 *Psychobiology is not an aetiological psychiatry, being content to remain on the descriptive level*
  Freudian mechanisms and Kraepelinian disease entities are both semantic illusions. Human behaviour cannot be reduced to absolute elements or essences.

3 *Psychobiology is superficial and never gets beneath into the zone of more significant action (ie. the unconscious)*
  This is the criticism from psychoanalysis, but psychiatric inquiry can be broadened when required to supplement what is immediately at hand. By contrast, special explanation and systematisation of the unconscious do not necessarily open up understanding and management, and can be counterproductive.

4 *Psychobiology is simply Kraepelinism parading in new language, and why learn new terms for old things?*
  Thinking dynamically and attempting to integrate behaviour completely should not be avoided because it is inconvenient, disturbing and requires more effort.

5 *Psychobiology is content with half-truths*
  The facts should be stated honestly rather than determined by professional security needs.

6 *Psychobiology's only distinctive offering is a philosophy of psychiatry. For actual work it depends on borrowings from other methods.*
  Actual method is different in practice, determined by its philosophy.

Treatment

I next want to look at the implications for treatment of the bio-psychological perspective. As may be imagined, Meyer concentrated on the personal element in treatment as well as diagnosis.

Treatment is not to be considered an attack on an impersonal 'disease entity'. Therapy is concerned with the mustering and offering of the best resources of adjustments and adaptations.

This means that the psychiatrist has a different role and function from specialists in other fields of medicine and surgery.

> The psychiatrist – the user of biography – must help the person himself transform the faulty and blundering attempt of nature to restore the balance, an attempt which has resulted in undermining the capacity for self-regulation.

The implication is the development of a focus on personal therapy, although, as previously discussed, not on psychoanalysis. Meyer's form of personal therapy has sometimes been called 'personality analysis'. However, this did not mean that social interventions were excluded. As mentioned previously, Meyer valued and encouraged the development of mental health social work and occupational therapy.

> Therapy is the systematic attempt to influence the future course of the event through the best use of available resources. The therapeutic situation is no wise to be construed as a closed-shop contract between physician and patient, to the exclusion of the interests of the environment.

This social sense promoted a constant need for determining the opportunities and the responsibilities of the person to society and society to the person. Again as previously mentioned, the promotion of mental hygiene goes beyond the bounds of personal responsibility and comes about because of the problems of mental health which society as a whole must assume.

In practice, Meyer distanced psychiatry from physical treatments by neglecting them. He refused to admit cases of general paresis because he regarded them as basically medical problems (Wortis, 1986). Essentially he regarded the advent of insulin shock therapy as a resurgence of medical emphasis where humane psychological interest should have prevailed. This did not mean that he did not respond to the hope of such physical treatments and in fact he advocated the experimental use of insulin shock therapy when it was first introduced.

As an illustration, a letter from William Alanson White to Meyer in 1936 asked Meyer for his views of the value of hypoglycaemic shock treatment in dementia praecox (Meyer Archives I/4025/9). White anticipated that Meyer might be conservatively minded toward the treatment. In fact, Meyer claimed that 'there is no doubt about the value of the attitude of seeking help on the part of the patient that gets stimulated', and felt 'not only justified but under obligation to give the matter a trial'. This generous attitude to the investigation of the treatment was clarified in a letter written a few weeks later to Joseph Wortis, who was the first American to become acquainted with the new insulin treatment of schizophrenia. In this letter (Meyer Archives I/4112/14), Meyer made a distinction between

> two extremes in the attempts to play the savior role in psychiatry: the work at the root – which is evidently *not* insulin work – and importations which have nothing specific to do with psychiatry but exploit the patient and resources through and for imported interests [his emphasis].

Meyer was always sorry to 'see the latter get on the top' and whenever it did, 'his interest waned'. Like the paresis problem, which he was willing to leave 'to the spirochaetist', as far as insulin treatment was concerned he thought he was dealing with 'even more of an importation apt to divert the attention completely from the illness by absorbing the attention in the direction of something pharmaceutical'.

Despite this aversion to biological treatments, Meyer's pluralism meant that he facilitated such developments, particularly by others. He did not oppose Henry Cotton's surgical programme to eliminate focal sepsis as the cause of mental illness (Scull, 2005). Nor was he antagonistic to lobotomy, instead being 'inclined to think that there are more possibilities in this operation than appear on the surface' (Freeman & Watts, 1950). He encouraged Walter Freeman, pioneer of the transorbital lobotomy, to 'follow up scrupulously the experience with each case', advice which Freeman pursued during his life with cross country trips to visit patients (El-Hai, 2005). Meyer had perhaps learnt the dangers of overstatement from the excesses of Henry Cotton. Nonetheless he suppressed a report of the poor outcome of Cotton's work in the forlorn hope that he could persuade Cotton to accept the reality of his results. Meyer seemed unable to appreciate the significant mutilations caused by overenthusiastic radical surgery.

The advantage of an enthusiasm for physical treatments is that it counters a therapeutic nihilism. However, the danger is that therapeutic zeal has led to justification of all sorts of groundless and sometimes damaging, if not lethal, medical interventions.

> There is nothing men will not do, there is nothing they have not done, to recover their health and save their lives. They have submitted to be half drowned in water, and half choked with gases, to be buried up to their chins in earth, to be seared with hot irons like galley slaves, to be

crimped with knives, like codfish, to have needles thrust into their flesh, and bonfires kindled on their skin, to swallow all sorts of abominations, and to pay for all this, as if blisters were a blessing and leeches were luxury. What more can be asked to prove their honesty and sincerity?

Oliver Wendell Holmes, quoted in Menninger, 1963

This *furor therapeuticus* needs to be restrained. This aim is implicit in psychobiology, even if Meyer did not always implement it in practice. I am not saying that sustaining hope is unimportant. Optimism implies faith in change and maintains motivation. Nonetheless, the need of the sick to be treated and the wish of the doctor to be able to provide that treatment must be constantly checked by self-criticism and controlled by valid evaluation of the evidence.

The remnants of the biopsychological approach

Brody (1994) describes the paradigm taught to his generation of psychiatric residents in the 1940s:

We understood mind and behaviour as contingent upon the brain, but our central therapeutic concern was with the life story of the individual patient interacting with others in the context of society and culture. Prolonged contact with individual patients and the meticulous study of their lives at varying phases in varying contexts influenced our thinking as scientists as well as clinicians. In particular, it emphasised the remarkable plasticity of human behaviour, and made us cautious about describing it in terms of the intrinsic nature of the person, rather than person-environment interaction. Classification (ie. diagnosis), thus, seemed less important as a final entity, a category into which individuals can be fitted than as a process, part of the effort to make a particular person's incomprehensible behaviour intelligible in terms of context as well as development, and allow it to be dealt with therapeutically.

This biopsychological consensus is less apparent now. Modern American psychiatry, studied by participant observation, appears to be 'of two minds', in that there is a divided consciousness created between the practices of drug therapy and psychotherapy (Luhrmann, 2000). Therapeutic advances in psychopharmacology since the introduction of chlorpromazine have served as the stimulus for biological theories (Sabshin, 1990). These have been reinforced by the development of brain imaging (Lieberman, 1999). Psychiatric diagnosis has became increasingly codified following the original paper by Feighner, et al (1972) and the introduction of the Research Diagnostic Criteria (Spitzer, et al, 1975), through editions of DSM-III, DSM-IIIR and DSM-IV (American Psychiatric Association, 1994). This explicit and intentional concern with psychiatric diagnosis, combined with a reinforcement of the biomedical model, contrasts with Meyer's views de-emphasising diagnosis in favour of understanding the life story of the individual patient.

Even though the biopsychological approach was never systematised as such, these recent biomedical developments have left the biopsychological approach even more disorganised. Strands may be detected since psychobiology and I want to briefly mention three of these.

William Alanson White (1933) played a major role in the introduction of psychoanalysis in the United States after 1910, advancing its role as a theory and treatment method. He was also mentor to Harry Stack Sullivan. The interpersonal approach of Sullivan focused on relationships and the effects of the individual's social and cultural environment on inner life (Barton Evans, 1996). Sullivan established the Washington School of Psychiatry (Rioch, 1986) in 1936 as the training institution of the William Alanson White Foundation. In the prospectus, Sullivan identified White, Meyer and A.A. Brill, translator of Freud and first American psycho-analyst, as the leaders of psychiatry. He invited Meyer to be lecturer with the rank of clinical professor in psychobiology in the new school, and then later to serve as honorary president after the death of White, which Meyer declined (Meyer Archives 1/3736/4). The Foundation established the journal *Psychiatry*, which Sullivan edited. A New York division of the school was organised under the leadership of Clara Thompson and in 1946 it gained a separate charter as the William Alanson White Institute. Erich Fromm joined Thompson, as did subsequently Harry Stack Sullivan, Freida Fromm-Reichmann and Janet and David Rioch. They formed an unusual alliance, based more on respect for freedom of thought and avoidance of dogma and idolatry than unanimity of perspective (Lionells, 2000). What they did agree on was the importance of interactions between individuals and their interpersonal environment. Sullivan, who died in 1949, was key to this perspective, although he was not as thoroughgoing in his biopsychological approach as Meyer and, for example, thought that the most degenerate forms of schizophrenia must have a biological cause. Nonetheless, these developments, epitomised by Sullivan, show a pluralism that is now less apparent in modern psychiatry, but is central to the biopsychological approach.

Another strand of the biopsychological approach comes from the relationship between anthropology and psychiatry because of the focus on culture. For example, Arthur Kleinman (1988) recognises the extent to which psychiatric diagnosis is a cultural judgement. He promotes a paradigm shift in medical and psychiatric practice to create a robust relationship between psychiatry and the social sciences. Similarly, Eisenberg (1986) encourages an integration of mind and body to avoid the 'mindlessness' of focusing exclusively on the brain as an organ and the 'brainlessness' of a psychodynamic psychotherapy which treats the brain sciences and empirical validation as irrelevant. Recent data on how experience moulds the brain holds out the possibility for mind–brain integration in the social construction of the brain (Eisenberg, 1995).

Thirdly, George Engel (1977) used general systems theory for his proposed biopsychosocial model, seen as a new challenge for bio-medicine. Perturbations occurring at any level in the hierarchical biopsychosocial system exert effects on other levels. The patient is conceptualised as being composed of systems (tissues, cells, molecules) and, in turn, as being part of several larger systems (dyads, families, communities, nations). McWhinney (1997) suggests that a paradigm shift in medicine will lead to the biopsychosocial model supplanting the anomalies of the biomedical model.

These three examples do not exhaust the representatives of the biopsychological perspective by any means, but are given here merely to illustrate its presence in psychiatry since Meyer.

Conclusion

My contention is that there has always been a biopsychological paradigm competing with the dominant biomedical model of mental illness. This trend began with Ernst von Feuchtersleben and was most identified with Adolf Meyer. Several strands can be identified since Meyer's time, but these have never been systematised or regarded as part of the mainstream of psychiatry. The biopsychological viewpoint has various assumptions (Wilson, 1993). Anyone can become mentally ill if exposed to sufficient trauma. The boundary between normality and insanity is relative rather than absolute. The cause of mental illness is postulated to be an untoward mixture of harmful environment and psychic conflict. Mental illness is conceived along a continuum of severity from neurosis through borderline conditions to psychosis. The mechanisms by which mental illness emerges in an individual are psychologically mediated. These points can be seen as the essential principles of the approach.

Despite the longevity of this perspective, it has always been a minority view and over recent years seems to have had even less of a voice. This may be because of its relation to anti-psychiatry. In some ways, the biopsychological perspective could be seen as the philosophical foundation underlying anti-psychiatry, at least the Laingian version. Anti-psychiatry had its excesses and is seen as unorthodox. Hence any attempt to restate the biopsychological model becomes tainted with the worst aspects of anti-psychiatry.

Furthermore, Meyer, despite being the most thoroughgoing representative of the paradigm failed, in his own words, 'to give real expression to my own trend' (Meyer Archives VI/8/199). In the heartfelt, early morning post-retirement note mentioned earlier, he questioned himself, 'Did I pussyfoot too much?' His tendency to compromise meant that his statements failed to be outspoken. By contrast, anti-psychiatry generated and thrived on the controversy it created.

As mentioned in chapter 1, there is a danger that the term 'critical psychiatry' may be understood as too oppositional. Nonetheless conflict maybe cannot be avoided in restating the biopsychological perspective in a post-anti-psychiatric age. Psychobiology was a valid viewpoint. There is as much of a consensus for the interpretative, biopsychological perspective as the biomedical model. It is just struggling to be restated after the turmoil caused by anti-psychiatry. The rest of this book together with this chapter is part of an attempt to create that new synthesis.

11

Critical Child Psychiatry

Sami Timimi

Introduction

Prescriptions of psychotropic medication to children and adolescents have shown a phenomenal increase in most Western countries (see below). To help understand how this came about, the cultural and political context that leads to medicalising social problems is examined. I propose that a perceived crisis of a social and moral nature, in Western countries, in relation to the cultural task of child rearing is an important factor behind this trend. Historically, the biggest changes in our beliefs about children and child rearing occur at times of perceived crises with regard to children. I argue that such a perceived crisis is occurring in Western society at present, creating favourable cultural conditions for the medicalisation of childhood problems, despite the lack of evidence to support such a construction. Looking at our changing constructions of childhood implies that the meaning we give to children's behaviour, changes over time (and is likely to continue to do so) making the idea that we know what a universal 'normal' childhood is, suspect. Given the political and economic power of Western states, there is a danger that ideas and practices we in the West are constructing are then being inappropriately exported worldwide. Thus a critical approach to understanding our professional practice requires us to consider the impact of our work on, not only the clients we see, but also on the broader culture locally and globally. Alternative approaches for practitioners are suggested.

Whilst these important contextual issues are beginning to receive attention in adult psychiatry, the debate on how such dynamics have affected child psychiatric practice is just beginning (Timimi, 2002a). Thus, the social control element of the rise in use of psychotropics for the purpose of behavioural control of children is only recently receiving some attention in mainstream journals (eg. Timimi & Taylor, 2004).

The social construction of childhood

To help us understand the context out of which child psychiatric beliefs and practices arose, we need to examine the cultural and political environment within which its institutions developed (Timimi, 2002a, 2005). This means examining our cultural beliefs on what constitutes a 'normal' childhood, from which, of course, our ideas concerning deviance are derived. Whilst the immaturity of children is a biological fact, the ways in which this immaturity is understood and made meaningful is a fact of culture (Prout & James, 1997). Members of any society carry within themselves a working definition of childhood, its nature, limitations and duration. They may not explicitly discuss this definition, write about it, or even consciously conceive of it as an issue, but they act upon their assumptions in all of their dealings with, fears for, and expectations of, their children (Calvert, 1992). Our construction of what makes a normal/pathological childhood is not 'innocent' of current political, economic, moral or indeed health concerns. Rather childhood often represents a central arena through which we construct our fantasies about the future and a battleground through which we struggle to express competing ideological agendas.

Thus our understanding of what makes a 'normal' or deviant childhood is socially constructed. For the sake of brevity and for its relevance to understanding the context out of which Western child psychiatry arises, I will limit myself to examining the West's changing views of childhood.

Western childhoods

Historians believe that modern, Western notions of childhood can be traced to the late 17th century when Locke published his influential *Some thoughts concerning education*. Locke proposed that children should be viewed as individuals waiting to be molded into shape by adults. In the mid-18th century, Rousseau published his highly influential *Emile* in which he argued that children were born with innate goodness that could be corrupted by certain kinds of education. These two books were crucial in paving the way for a new focus, in European culture, on childhood, which was now being viewed as requiring separate needs/expectations than adulthood. By the mid-19th century, childhood was viewed as a distinct entity requiring protection and fostering through school education. Using the perceived social crisis of the time, the ruling classes used these new values to paint working-class children as the source of many social problems and as children neglected by their parents who, as a result, were potentially dangerous future juvenile delinquents and criminals. This helped smooth the way for mass education and helped prepare public opinion, for introducing the state into the parent/child relationship (Hendrick, 1997).

By the beginning of the 20th century children in Western, capitalist states were seen as individuals on whom the state could have a more fundamental influence than their families. Now that children were all in schools they also became readily available to a variety of professionals for all sorts of 'scientific' surveys. Professional interest in the idea of child development grew and the scientific study of the individual child was encouraged in an effort to produce 'guiding principles' to be offered to parents and teachers. The medical and psychological professions helped popularise the view that childhood is marked by stages in normal development. A number of assumptions derived from psycho-medicine about what constituted normal childhood development and normal parenting were made. At the same time the state was becoming more interventionist through legislation following a debate about children's rights and an assumption that only the state could enforce these rights (Hendrick, 1997).

Before the onset of the Second World War, Western society viewed relations between parents and children primarily in terms of discipline and authority. This pre-war paradigm, grounded in behaviourism, stressed the importance of forming habits of behaviour necessary for productive life. During the Second World War anxiety about the impact on children of discipline and authority began to be expressed, the concern being that 'despotic' discipline could lead to the sort of nightmare society that Nazi Germany represented. Scholarly and professional discourses that spoke about the child as an individual and which favoured a more democratic approach to child rearing, encouraging humane discipline of the child through guidance and understanding, helped popularise new ideals, eventually resulting in the birth of the 'permissive' culture (Jenkins, 1998). The 'permissiveness' model saw parent–child relations increasingly in terms of pleasure and play. Parents now had to relinquish traditional authority in order for children to develop autonomy and self-worth. In addition, whilst the pre-war model prepared children for the workplace within a society of scarcity, the post-war model prepared them to become pleasure-seeking consumers within a prosperous new economy (Wolfenstein, 1955).

Childhood, through a process of miniaturization, became a key metaphor through which adults spoke about their social and political concerns. Thus permissiveness with regards to child rearing was allowing,

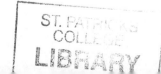

not only, new identities to be prescribed for children, but also for adults. Mothers and fathers were responding to this changing definition of childhood and seeing this as a vehicle for fuller expression for them. Parental obligations were paving the way for the culture of fun and permissiveness for all.

Following the traumas of the Second World War and the evacuation process for children in Britain, prominence was also given to the effects of early separation of young children from their mothers. This construction was reinforced by the development of attachment theory by the British psychoanalyst John Bowlby (1969, 1973). Separation, it was now claimed, produced an affectionless character that was the root cause of anti-social behaviour (Bowlby, 1969, 1973).

Shifting economic structures were also leading to profound changes in the organisation of family life. More mothers were working and thus a renegotiation of power within the family was taking place. Suburbanization and the economic demands of successful market economies were resulting in greater mobility, less time for family life and a breakdown of the extended family. Many families (particularly those headed by young women) were now isolated from traditional sources of child rearing information. In this context child rearing guides took on an unprecedented importance allowing for a more dramatic change in parenting styles than would have been conceivable in a more rooted community, and greater 'ownership' by professionals of the knowledge base for the task of parenting (Zuckerman, 1975).

The new child-centred permissive culture was a godsend to consumer capitalism, and an industry of children's toys, books, fun educational material and so on developed (Weinman-Lear, 1963). The culture of consumption (with its expectations of a 'fun morality') became a major force shaping child-rearing practices of the 20th century in the West. With the expansion of the consumer marketplace and suburban affluence, permissive conceptions of the child embraced pleasure as a positive motivation for exploration and learning.

Although a backlash against the culture of permissiveness took place particularly in the 1980s and 90s, it was already embedded in modern Western notions of childhood, put the individual at the centre, and was in the service of capital following a period of decline in western economies. More parents were forced to work for longer hours, and state support particularly for children and families was harshly cut resulting in widespread child poverty and the creation of a new under-class.

With the increase in the number of divorces and two working parents, fathers and mothers are around their children for less of the day. As kids are forced to withdraw into their own culture the free market exploits this, praying on their boredom and desire for stimulation (Kincheloe, 1998). In this environment poor children are constantly confronted with their shortcomings by media that tells them they are deficient without this or that accessory. In this unhappy isolation Western children respond to the markets push to 'adultify' them (at the same time as the culture of self-gratification 'childify's' adults) by entering into the world of adult entertainments earlier and without adult supervision. Thus the postmodern Western child is sexually knowledgeable and has early experience of drugs and alcohol (Aronowitz & Giroux, 1991). Many argue that as a result childhood in the West is being eroded, lost or indeed is suffering a strange death (Jenhs, 1996). It is claimed that childhood is disappearing as children have gained access to the world of adult information resulting in a blurring of boundaries between what is considered adulthood and what is considered childhood, leading to children coming to be viewed as in effect miniature adults. In such a context the idea of 'childhood innocence' comes to be viewed nostalgically, as something belonging to the past, an idea that many politicians from a variety of persuasions then use for their own purposes (for example to talk about returning to traditional family values) (Jenkins, 1998).

One result of these competing discourses and changes in family and lifestyle has been the development of some core tensions and ambivalence with regard to children. The children's rights movements, see childhood as being at risk and needing safeguarding against pollution by adults (often without noticing how much the permissive, children's rights discourse has already eroded boundaries between adults and children), whilst simultaneously seeing childhood as needing strengthening by developing children's character and ability to reason. In other words, on the one hand childhood needs to be preserved and on the other hand it is made older than its years. This contradiction runs through our modern conception of childhood innocence, we desire it and we want to help children to move beyond it, we want to 'coddle' the child and we want to 'discipline' the child (Aries, 1998).

At the same time there has been a growing concern that children themselves have become the danger with children being viewed as deviant and violent troublemakers despite coming from a generation who are perceived to have been given the best of everything (Seabrook, 1982; Alcock & Harris, 1982). Thus by the end of the 20th century our vision of childhood in the West is a polarised one, at one pole we have victimised 'innocent' children who need rescuing, at the other pole we have impulsive, aggressive, sexual children who are a threat to society. Just as children are polarised, so are parents who are now set impossible standards by the child savers, many finding themselves marginalised, as potentially abusive parents, by child welfare professionals (Scheper-Hughes & Stein, 1987). Being viewed as a 'normal' child and a 'normal' parent has arguably, become, harder than ever to achieve.

The common thread through both these visions of 'childhood at risk' and 'children as the risk' is the suggestion that modern society has seen a collapse of adult authority (morally and physically). This collapse is reflected in the growth in parental spending on children and the endless search by parents for emotional gratification for their children (Cunningham, 1995; Zelizer, 1985). As increasing concerns are voiced about children's development, so fingers have pointed towards the role of the family, particularly mothers, the genetic make-up of the child and the nature of schooling environments. Judgements about abnormal childhoods and family forms have become harsher; such that parents and children feel ever more closely scrutinised (Boyden, 1997; Winn, 1984; Morgan, 1987; Barlow & Hill, 1985).

Whilst parents are feeling the pressure to constantly scrutinise their practices in order to measure up to the high expectations from the authority breakdown discourse and to quell the anxiety from the child welfare discourse, schools have also had to respond to these dual pressures. The result at the individual child level has been a mushrooming of individual child explanations, locating the cause of the anxiety within individual children and resulting in the development of a new reconstruction of childhood in primarily biological/genetic terms.

The medicalisation of childhood

With the medical profession having played a central role in developing modern, Western ideas about child development and child rearing, it has been ideally placed both socially and politically, to respond to this cultural anxiety. Using its status and position of power to further increase its own influence over children and families, paediatrics, child psychiatrists and psychologists have chosen popular post-European enlightenment cultural preoccupations with reason and the individual subject, as well as being subject to the same market demands of increasing personal profitability. Thus context deprived approaches that focus on the individual child, as the locus of this anxiety, with the idea that a chemical imbalance or neurological delay in development is the cause of a child's perceived problems, has become commonplace practice in the West. As with adult psychiatry no evidence of pathological lesions has been forthcoming and there are no neurological, psychological or other physical markers to assist the clinician in making childhood and adolescent psychiatric disorder diagnosis. The question of the validity of conceptualizing the new concepts (such as attention deficit hyperactivity disorder, Aspergers syndrome, childhood depression) within a medical framework has been largely avoided.

Market economies need to continually expand markets has allowed drug companies to exploit these new, vague and broadly defined childhood psychiatric diagnoses, resulting in a rapid increase in the amount of psychotropic medication being prescribed to children and adolescents in the West. For example, the amount of psychotropic medication prescribed to children in the United States increased nearly four fold between 1985 and 1994 (Pincus et al, 1998). More recently researchers analysing prescribing trends in nine countries (UK, France, Germany, Spain, Canada, USA, Argentina, Brazil, and Mexico), between 2000 and 2002, found that significant rises in the number of prescriptions for psychotropic drugs in children, were evident in all countries – the lowest being in Germany where the increase was 13 per cent, and the highest being in the UK where an increase of 68 per cent was recorded (Wong et al, 2004). Little research has been done on the safety and efficacy of psychotropic drugs in children, with prescribing patterns in children often being based on information drawn from research in adults. Of particular concern is the increase in rates of stimulant prescription to children. By 1996 over 6% of school-aged boys in America were taking stimulant medication (Olfson et al, 2002) with children as young as two being prescribed stimulants in increasing numbers (Zito et al, 2000). Recent surveys show that in some schools in the United States over 17% of boys are taking stimulant medication (LeFever et al, 1999). In the UK prescriptions for stimulants have increased from about 6,000 in 1994 to about 345,000 children in the latter half of 2003 (Wright, 2003), suggesting that we in the UK are rapidly catching up with the US.

With enormous profits to be made for the pharmaceutical industry, the combination of doctors carving out new and increasing roles for themselves together with aggressive marketing by the drug industry, a very powerful and difficult to resist combination has arisen. Privileged social groups, who hold important and influential positions, have a powerful effect on our common cultural beliefs, attitudes and practices. Child psychiatry in the UK does appear to have re-invented itself in the last ten years. Influential child psychiatrists successfully influenced the UK's professional discourse convincing it that there were more personal rewards for the profession by it adopting a more medicalised American style approach (eg. Goodman, 1997). This has encouraged not only, the creation and widespread 'recognition' for new child psychiatric diagnoses but also the construction of whole new classes of disorder – such as 'neuro-developmental psychiatry', which the public, trusting such high status opinions, has come to view as real.

Modern child psychiatric practice is now characterized by symptom based, context deprived assessments, use of screening questionnaires, aggressive use of psychotropic medication and use of multiple prescriptions often with little information about safety or long-term consequences (Pincus et al, 1998). As with adult psychiatry this places child psychiatry in a symbiotic discourse with the political establishment. Not only do we continue to make fundamental contributions to everyday thinking about what is normal and abnormal for children and parenting, but we also volunteer ourselves as powerful agents of social control.

A critique of the evidence supporting a biomedical model; two case examples

Attention Deficit Hyperactivity Disorder (ADHD)

There are no specific cognitive, metabolic or neurological markers for ADHD. Those who have argued that ADHD does not exist as a real disorder, start by pointing to the obvious uncertainty about its definition (McGuinness, 1989). Because of this uncertainty epidemiological studies have produced very different prevalence rates for ADHD (in its various forms), ranging from about 0.5 per cent of school age children to 26 per cent of school age children (Taylor & Hemsley, 1995; Green et al, 1999).

Despite attempts at standardising criteria and assessment tools in cross-cultural studies, major and significant differences between raters from different countries continue to be apparent (Mann et al, 1992). There are also significant differences between raters when raters rate children from different ethnic minority backgrounds (Sonuga-Barke et al, 1993). One replicated finding is an apparently high rate of hyperactivity in China and Hong Kong (Shen et al, 1985; Luk & Leung, 1989). In these studies nearly three times as many Chinese as English children were rated as hyperactive. A more detailed assessment of these results suggested that most of the 'hyperactive' Chinese children would not have been rated as hyperactive by most English raters and were a good deal less hyperactive than English children rated as 'hyperactive' (Taylor, 1994), thus demonstrating that hyperactivity and disruptiveness (particularly in boys) is a highly culturally constructed entity.

That ratings of hyperactivity, inattention and disruptiveness are culturally dependent is not surprising as inattention, impulsivity and motor restlessness are found in all children (and adults) to some degree. Diagnosis is based on an assessment of what is felt to be developmentally inappropriate intensity, frequency and duration of the behaviours, rather than on its mere presence. All the symptoms described in this disorder are of a subjective nature (eg. 'often does not seem to listen when spoken to') and therefore highly influenced by the raters cultural beliefs and perceptions about such behaviours. After all how do you operationalise, define and understand non-specific words like 'often' and 'excessive', which are invariably found in ADHD rating questionnaires?

Numerous epidemiological and clinical studies demonstrate the high frequency with which supposedly separate child psychiatric disorders occur in individuals with ADHD (Caron & Rutter, 1991). In children diagnosed with ADHD co-morbidity with other child psychiatric conditions is common no matter what definition is used (Beiderman et al, 1991). The co-occurrence of the symptoms that make up oppositional/defiant and conduct disorders with those that make up hyperactivity and attention deficit disorders is so strong (Beiderman et al, 1991; Fergusson & Horwood, 1993) that many commentators have questioned the reality of the distinction between them. Psychiatrists have adopted co-morbidity as a way of trying to explain clinical reality when it does not appear to tally with research generated views of mental life. It's a way of maintaining a fantasy that there is a natural, probably biological, boundary where no natural boundaries exist (Tyrer, 1996).

Claims have been made that neuroimaging studies confirm that ADHD is a brain disorder. Closer examination of the quoted studies not only reveals a more complex picture, it actually suggests the opposite, as the studies demonstrate that there is no characteristic neurophysiological or neuroanatomical pattern that can be found in children diagnosed as having ADHD. In no study have the brains of the ADHD diagnosed children been considered to be clinically abnormal (Hynd & Hooper, 1995), nor has any specific abnormality been convincingly demonstrated (Baumeister & Hawkins, 2001). Interestingly, after almost twenty-five years and over thirty such studies, researchers have yet to do a simple comparison of unmedicated children diagnosed with ADHD with an age matched control group, with the one large study that claimed to have done this (Castellanos et al, 2002) choosing a control group whose age was on average two years older (Leo & Cohen, 2003) and thereby all they scientifically managed to prove was that younger children had smaller brains than older ones! Most worryingly, animal studies suggest that any differences observed in these studies could well be due to the effects of medication that most children in these studies had taken (Breggin, 1999, 2001; Moll et al, 2001; Sproson et al, 2001).

What we end up with is speculative 'biobabble'. Even if consistent differences in neuroimaging studies were found, unidirectional cause and effect cannot be assumed. This is because neurophysiological measures may reflect different children's different reaction to the same situation causing differences in brain chemistry rather than different brain chemistry causing different behaviour (Christie et al, 1995). Thus, differences in brain function have been demonstrated in normal healthy children who have different temperaments (Fox et al, 1995).

In the rest of medicine, what has made diagnosis a useful way of categorising health problems, is that the diagnoses point to unique aetiological processes. In ADHD no unique aetiological processes have been identified. Indeed, the National Institute of Health, a government body in the United States, concluded that there is no evidence to support the proposition that ADHD is a biological brain disorder (National Institutes of Health, 1998). This conclusion is further supported by a large body of family, twin and adoption studies that support the idea that a genetic component contributes to hyperactivity, conduct disorder and other externalising behaviours in a manner that suggests a common genetic mechanism underlies all these disorders (Timimi, 2002a; Silberg et al, 1996). Presumably this common genetic mechanism has something to do with being a boy (boys are three to ten times more likely to be diagnosed with ADHD). As with neuroimaging as soon as ADHD supporters focus on specifics, their argument starts to fall apart. Thus Schachar & Tannock (2002) argue that molecular genetic variations have been robustly re-plicated, concluding that ADHD is associated with the dopamine transporter gene (DAT1) and the dopamine receptor gene (D4); yet a recent study of 126 sibling pairs concluded that these two genes if they are involved in ADHD aetiology at all, make only a minor contribution to overall genetic susceptibility (Fisher et al, 2002).

If instead we assume that behaviours such as motor activity, attention and impulsivity are normally distributed temperamental characteristics, then the evidence makes more sense. Research on children's temperament has shown that problems result from a mismatch between the child's temperament and their environment (Thomas & Chess, 1977; Chess & Thomas, 1996). Even children who are highly difficult temperamentally can become well adjusted behaviourally if their family and other social circumstances are supportive (Mazaide, 1989). One interpretation of this evidence is that behaviours we call ADHD are probably inherited in much the same way as other personality traits, whether these behaviours come to be perceived as a problem is mediated by psychosocial factors and the meaning we give them.

The popularity of the ADHD diagnosis has been further strengthened through interest in the merits of prescribing stimulant medication to children. Stimulants central nervous systems effects are not limited to those children who can be defined by the boundaries of this disorder.

Thus stimulants have the same cognitive and behavioural effects on otherwise normal children (Rapoport et al, 1978, 1980; Garber et al, 1996), aggressive children regardless of diagnosis (Spencer et al, 1996) and children with co-morbid conduct disorder (Taylor et al, 1987; Spencer et al, 1996). This is not surprising. The pharmacological action of stimulants on the brain is basically that of amphetamines (or its street name – speed) and cocaine (Volkow et al, 1995), which is known to have similar effects on most people who take it.

Research on treatment of ADHD with stimulants (like Ritalin) has focused almost exclusively on short-term outcomes. Outcome research in stimulant treatment has been shown to have serious shortfalls in methodology such as small samples, inadequate description of randomisation or blinding and not accounting for withdrawals or drop outs (Zwi et al, 2000; Joughin & Zwi, 1999). A recent meta-analysis of randomised controlled trials of methylphenidate found that the trials were of poor quality, there was strong evidence of publication bias, short-term effects were inconsistent across different rating scales, side effects were frequent and problematic and long-term effects beyond four weeks of treatment were not demonstrated (Schachter et al, 2001). The MTA group study (1999) has been highly influential and set a dangerous precedent in its conclusion that medication is better than psychosocial therapies. This study has been widely criticised on many grounds including; lack of placebo group or blinding, authors being firm advocates of ADHD and well known recipients of drug company money, playing down of the numbers of children experiencing side effects, participants already being 'cultured' into believing the children involved had a biological condition, study only lasting 14 months, and the fact that two thirds of those in the poorest outcome group (community treatment) were taking the very same stimulants. The few long-term studies that have been conducted suggest that stimulants do not result in any long-term improvement in either behavioural or academic achievement (Weis et al, 1975; Rie et al, 1976; Charles & Schain, 1981; Gadow, 1983; Hetchman et al, 1984; Klein & Mannuzza, 1991). Despite the lack of evidence for any long-term effectiveness, Ritalin is most usually prescribed continuously for seven, eight or more years, with children as young as two being prescribed the drug in increasing numbers despite the manufacturers licence stating that it should not be prescribed to children under six (Zito et al, 2000; Baldwin & Anderson, 2000).

Ritalin is also a drug of abuse as it can be crushed and snorted to produce a high (Heyman, 1994). Surveys have shown that a significant proportion of adolescents in the United States self report using Ritalin for non-medical purposes (Robin & Barkley, 1998). Accounts of abuse of

Ritalin and other stimulants are increasingly being reported in the lay press (Ravenel, 2002). A national survey in the United States found that 2.8 per cent of high school seniors had used Ritalin without a physician's prescription during the previous year (Sannerud & Feussner, 2000). The neuro-chemical effects of Ritalin are very similar to that of cocaine, which is one of the most addictive drugs. Cocaine users report that the effect of injected Ritalin is almost indistinguishable from that of cocaine (Volkow et al, 1995). A large community based study (Lambert & Hartsough, 1998) has found a significant increase in cocaine and tobacco dependence amongst ADHD subjects prescribed stimulants when compared to controls; furthermore, they discovered a linear relationship between the amount of stimulant treatment and the likelihood of either tobacco or cocaine dependence in later life. Ritalin remains a controversial drug for reasons that go well beyond its side effects. Yet these issues that should be important information for all parents trying to make the difficult decision as to whether or not to agree for their children to take a stimulant is information that is rarely given by prescribers (Baldwin & Cooper, 2000)

Childhood depression

According to the current criteria, psychiatric co-morbidity in childhood depression is so high nearly every child can be diagnosed with at least one other psychiatric condition (Harrington, 1994), raising the same doubts as ADHD with regard the specificity of the construct. Despite awareness of the continuity between normal sadness and clinical depression, the diagnosis assumes that clinical depression exists as a category (rather than on a continuum). It is unclear, however, who decides where the cut-off mark is, and on what basis.

Furthermore, the categorical diagnosis bears only a tenuous relation with levels of psychosocial impairment. Many children below the threshold of diagnosis show higher levels of impairment than those above the threshold (Pickles et al, 2001). Similarly, a diagnosis of childhood depression is only weakly associated with suicide (stronger predictors include history of aggression and use of drugs or alcohol) (Wickes-Nelson & Israel, 2002). The biological markers (such as dexamethasone suppression of cortisol) that are sometimes found in adults diagnosed with depression do not work with children and adolescents diagnosed as depressed (Harrington, 1994). With regards to genetics, separating environmental from biological factors in the familial clustering has been virtually impossible, particularly as children whose parents have depression are at risk of developing a wide range of psychiatric disorders (Wickes-Nelson & Israel, 2002).

Childhood depression has been argued to be a precursor of adulthood depression (Harrington et al, 1993). However, follow up studies of children deemed to have had 'major depressive disorders' have used dubious standards for diagnosing childhood and adult psychiatric disorders, have discovered high rates of co-morbidity (in childhood and adulthood), have been unable to differentiate biological factors from continuing social adversity (Harrington et al, 1993; Fombonne et al, 2001), and have not taken into account the possible effects of any treatment received (such as continuing morbidity as a result of toxic side effects of drug treatment and the experience of psychosocial adversity and decreased self worth arising from becoming a psychiatric patient).

Leading researchers claim that childhood depression resembles adult depression (Harrington, 1994). However, based on symptoms alone, children do not show many of the symptoms said to be common in adult depression (such as loss of weight and appetite, sleep disturbance, and feelings of guilt). Instead more non-specific symptoms such as irritability, running away from home, decline in schoolwork, and headaches are described as indicative of childhood depression (Hill, 1997).

Despite its poor evidence base, the concept of 'childhood depression' has become commonplace causing a shift in theory, and consequently practice, toward a context depleted interpretation of the meaning behind childhood unhappiness. The medicalisation of childhood unhappiness has in turn resulted in antidepressants often becoming a first line treatment (Jureidini et al, 2004a), despite antidepressants being largely ineffective in the under-18s with the potential to cause serious side effects (Timimi, 2004; Jureidini et al, 2004a, b).

The implication for children and society

Without good evidence to support the idea that these new diagnoses are the result of physical pathology, the medicalisation of the West's views on child development and child rearing, is best understood as the West's most recent way of interpreting how children should be, rather than the result of scientific endeavour that is leading us ever closer to the 'truth' about the universal nature of childhood. Just as we may look back with a critical eye at previous generations' assumptions about the nature of child development, there is no reason to assume that we have reached some final end-point in our current assumptions, and that we will not similarly be criticised by future generations. To conclude that our current Western views of child development are socially constructed (in other words we are creating not discovering the meanings we give to children's behaviour and emotional state) is not enough; we still have to critique the utility to children, families, and society of the preferred meanings we give.

Within Western child developmental discourse there is a constant subtext that is saying there is a superior and inferior position. Development says to the child, the parent and the teacher this is your future and if you do not reach it you are, in some senses, inferior (Morss, 1996). It is not just children who are said to develop but also peoples and economies (Rahman, 1993; Sachs, 1992). Development is about modern hierarchies of superiority and inferiority – it is about dismissing diversity. Developmental explanations instil the notion of individual competitiveness; from the moment you are born you will have developmental milestones thrust upon you. As parents we are desperate to see our children achieve these age bound expectations. Development of our children is under constant professional surveillance starting with health visitors and community paediatricians and moving on to general practitioners, nursery nurses, teachers and the whole range of para-psycho-medicine specialists. We are concerned when our children seem to be falling behind and we are constantly encouraging them to achieve these expectations. If we are not concerned and not encouraging, presumably we are neglecting.

And what of the children themselves? If there is a belief that these are natural, unfolding processes for which professionals must be involved in helping children achieve, does this not encourage competitiveness from a very early age? How much do children get caught in these parental and professional anxieties? How relaxed can children, from the moment they are born, be to just be, as opposed to having to do something to ease these cultural anxieties? When these anxieties cannot be comforted and there is a perception that a child has strayed from their pre-destined development path, who is to blame? In this blame-ridden culture that needs an explanation for everything much of the developmental psychopathology literature has generally pointed toward the mother for blame and more recently toward the child's genes. In a culture where families have shrunk and fathers seem to disappear and relinquish duty and responsibility in ever increasing numbers, mothers often have to shoulder not only the responsibility for caring for their family (a role given much lower status in Western culture than many non-Western cultures), but also for things going wrong. In a final stab from the developmental discourse mothers are then denied credit for their work when things do go well as children are then simply seen as achieving their biological destiny.

Within this context the more bio-deterministic aspects of the developmental and developmental psychopathology culture has, at least, appeared to provide a get-out clause for the beleaguered mother. Now problems can be viewed as being the result of a fault in the genetic programme for development and thus intrinsic to the child. But this approach to understanding the problems of children is equally guilty in its simplistic theoretical assumptions, and in denying alternative possibilities. Furthermore, it never solves the nagging doubt in the back of a parent's mind that it is their fault, leads to children internalising a potentially lifelong personal script of disability (with its potential for disconnecting a person from their own capacity for agency), and exposes children to a plethora of untested, possibly harmful, psychotropic medications.

Western child development/psychiatric disorder beliefs heavily influence the education system our children grow up in. For example the defining of a disability requiring special needs help at school is shaped by the disciplines of medicine and psychology (Hey et al, 1998). The adherence of these two fields to measuring physical and mental competence in order to determine normality inevitably conveys assumptions about deviance and failure and these labels then become attached to both individuals and groups which have failed to measure up/conform. Special needs practice within schools rests on within child explanations (Ainscow & Tweddle, 1988) and on the whole are focused upon reading ability or acting out behaviour (or naughtiness) (Daniels et al, 1998). There are important gender differences with special needs resources in schools going to a much higher proportion of boys than girls (Daniels et al, 1998). There are also obvious differences in special needs provision within schools by race, with black pupils appearing to be systematically diverted from the category of specific reading difficulties and allocated to mild to moderate learning difficulties and black boys in particular to emotional and behavioural difficulties, while white boys tend to dominate the reading support resources (Hey et al, 1998). Like the professions of psychology and psychiatry, teaching has fallen victim of rationalist, scientific, market values and has moved toward a more 'technicist' approach, with greater emphasis on specialisation and less acknowledgement of the human social exchange nature of a teacher's activity, leading to: deskilling and greater emotional detachment from their work (Skelton, 2001), the return of more didactic beliefs and practices in school that revolve around concepts derived from a child development perspective, and an increase in the number of children referred by schools for medical management (usually with medication) of behaviour problems (Timimi, 2005).

Then there is the problem of colonialism. Western attitudes and beliefs with regard to child rearing are being exported to countries conceptualised as 'underdeveloped' (in moral/ethical/knowledge as well as economic spheres) and taken up by local professionals many of whom understandably believe they are getting something better from the more sophisticated and advanced West. For example the *Handbook of Asian child development and child rearing practices* (Suvannathat, 1985), prepared by Thai child development experts, is highly influenced by Western medico-psychological ideology. The book sets out to assimilate Western child development theory into a third world context with very little evidence of taking a local perspective into account. Thus the authors suggest that many of the traditional beliefs and practices of Asians prevent them from seeking and using new scientific knowledge in child rearing, and go on to argue, in line with Western thinking, that children should be given more independence with less use of power and authority by the parents.

Just as problematic notions of child rearing are being imposed on countries of the South, so also are problematic notions of child mental health problems. Economically and politically powerful groups, such as the doctors and the pharmaceutical industry, have enabled Western medicine to push back its frontiers of influence. Rapid growth in the prescribing of psychotropic medications to children is happening in many countries of the South (such as Brazil and Mexico) (Wong et al, 2004), suggesting the Western individualised biological/genetic conception of childhood mental health problems is spreading to the countries of the South and may be undermining more helpful indigenous belief systems with regard the problems of childhood (Timimi, 2002a, b, 2005).

The current trend for medicalising childhood also reminds us of the values behind the eugenic movement. Human experience deprived of context and examined through the prism of apparent scientific objectivity lends itself perfectly to being used by the political system of the day (Timimi, 2002a). Medical concepts of mental illness naturally focus on individuals' differences and perceived inadequacies when compared to the cultural norm. With the absence of 'treatments' that return a deviant group back into the desired cultural norm, together with the embedded idea that these deviants are corrupted with poor genes, makes it a short step to proposing eugenic solutions for this perceived 'medical' problem. Medical practitioners can then excuse their actions by believing that they are participating in a 'treatment' that is for the good of the future medical well-being of society. Once we have defined our perception of what we consider to be socially deviant as being caused by a medical disorder, it is only a short step towards the idea of preventing these behaviours from happening in the first place by use of medical means (Harper & Clarke, 1997). Thus psychiatrists involved in exterminating psychiatric inpatients at the beginning of the Nazi's eugenic programme, did not merely supervise, but it was often the duty of a psychiatrist to open the valve of the cylinder containing the carbon monoxide as if they were supervising a treatment (Muller-Hill, 1991). In 2004, the Bush government announced plans for a national screening programme where it aims to screen all children for signs of psychiatric disorder, a plan that cynics rightly condemn as an attempt to help the pharmaceutical industry fish for new customers (Lenzer, 2004), but also suggests a worrying trend toward greater medicalisation of social issues, a trend that could lead to eugenic ideals re-entering into our modern cultural discourse.

A multi-perspective approach to child psychiatry

Is it possible to progress practice in this area in a way that is mindful of these context issues? It is always difficult to promote non-mainstream practice. To do so in a way that affects everyday clinical practice in a meaningful way often requires us to embrace a mindset of openness and acceptance of diversity. Developing interventions that are mindful of the political and cultural dynamics I discuss above can be thought of at three different levels (Timimi, 2002a, 2005):

The work of culture in defining a problem

Different cultures see different behaviours as problematic. For example, when Western culture is compared to many other cultures, we notice that in many non-Western cultures fewer expectations are placed on infants and younger children with regards to their behaviour, emotional expression and self-control, but older children are expected to accept 'adult' responsibilities earlier. A model of child development that recognises that different cultures have different equally healthy versions of child development has the potential to reduce the amount of pathologising of childhood that currently occurs in Western medical practice. This would mean the profession actively engaging in questioning the universal validity of the concepts and rating questionnaires used.

Different cultures use different approaches to solve problems

Within Western culture as well as medication, there are other therapeutic modalities that can be helpfully used, such as family therapy, cognitive behavioural therapy and psychodynamic psychotherapy. In addition, it should be recognised that all communities have resources, whether that is within the immediate family, extended family, religious community, schools and other institutions, that may well have positive suggestions and interventions to offer. For many non-Western cultures, the family not the individual is regarded as the basic social unit. Family's strengths can be recognised and promoted. A spiritual dimension may also be important and can be explored. Ideas from other systems of medicine can be utilised. For example Ayurvedic medicine sees illness as a disruption in the delicate somatic, climactic and social system of balance. Causes are not located as such but seen as part of a system out of balance with symptoms viewed as being a part of a process rather than a disease entity (Obeyesekere, 1977). Such an attitude based on balance with nature (as opposed to controlling it) has resonance with new approaches that include lifestyle interventions focusing on aspects such as diet, exercise and family routines (Timimi, 2005).

Different culture's beliefs, values and practices promote and curtail certain types of behaviours and experiences

The rise in the rates of prescription of psychotropic medication for children and adolescents may also be the result of an increase in what might be loosely termed psychosocial suffering amongst children in Western society (Timimi, 2004, 2005). This may have something to do with the cultural experiences of children. As socially respected practitioners, we have a responsibility to understand that we bring a cultural value system into our work. We cannot be dispassionate bystanders. Our actions will ripple out into the wider local community. We need to consider the ethics of our actions and be able to take a long-term socially responsible perspective. With regard to policy we could campaign for more family friendly policies such as fighting global child poverty, family friendly business practices, and criminalising willfully absent parents.

Conclusion

12

Critical Psychiatry and Conflict: Renewing Mental Health Practice

D.B. Double

One of Donald Kiesler's conclusions in his book *Beyond the disease model of mental disorders* is that, 'We have to stop acquiescing to pontifications that mental disorders are brain diseases' (Kiesler 1999: 199). He argues that all educated lay persons and scientists of psychopathology must quit professing, or tolerating others who advocate or imply, single causes of mental disorder.

Kiesler's stance should be applauded. However, it may also be seen as too confrontational. The chapters in this book have reinforced his conclusion about the nature of mental disorder. As I mentioned in my chapter on the biopsychological approach (chapter 11), Adolf Meyer towards the end of his life questioned whether he had been outspoken enough about psychobiology. He wondered to himself, 'Did I pussyfoot too much? [in getting his message across]'. The danger of trying to accommodate all perspectives, as Meyer attempted to do, is that Meyerian psychiatry could be said to have become 'intellectually empty' and 'ethically blind', and this is, for example, Andrew Scull's (2005) verdict. There is a fine balance to be drawn between polarising the debate about the nature of mental illness, of which anti-psychiatry stands accused, and being assertive enough to avoid overcompromising on principles.

However admirable Kiesler's intentions may be, we also may have to be realistic that there is unlikely to be a radical paradigmatic shift in psychiatric practice. The biomedical model of mental illness is too well entrenched. However vehemently the biomedical model is opposed, it will defend itself and fortify its position. It has an assured authority that does not easily surrender to challenge. It has been ascendant ever since the beginnings of modern psychiatry in the mid-19th century.

Mental health work has always generated controversial issues in thought and practice (Clare, 1980). There may be less debate now about these issues than previously. An eclectic consensus could be said to have settled from the fall-out of 'anti-psychiatry'. Critical psychiatry does not want to disrupt this sense of harmony for its own sake. However, it is looking for a new synthesis. Critical psychiatry agrees with 'anti-psychiatry' that social processes, such as psychiatric practice, require continuous critical assessment. Mainstream psychiatric theory still has the mistaken tendency, for which it was attacked by anti-psychiatry, of relying on unfounded speculations about the nature of mental illness. Although biomedical psychiatry may wish itself to be a simple, straightforward, scientific discipline, in fact its ideological nature and its relationship to issues of power are unavoidable.

By way of concluding this book, I want briefly, in general terms, to summarise and attempt to define critical psychiatry, describe the key issues and clarify how critical psychiatry differs from mainstream psychiatry. These issues have been taken up generally and in places in more detail in the rest of the chapters of the book, but it may be helpful to reiterate them for the purpose of clarification.

The nature of critical psychiatry

(i) *What is critical psychiatry?*

Critical psychiatry is the name for an approach that encourages a self-critical attitude to psychiatric practice. An adverse consequence of the term 'critical' is that it tends to have a negative connotation. In this sense, 'critical' means 'inclined to find fault, or to judge with severity'. However, 'critical' also has other meanings, such as being 'characterised by careful, exact evaluation and judgement'. Also, it may have something to do with a crucial turning point, in this sense meaning 'of the greatest importance to the way things might happen'. These latter senses are included in the way I am using the word 'critical' in relation to psychiatry.

I want to suggest that the essence of critical psychiatry can be looked at from three related perspectives. These are (a) its relationship to critical thinking (b) its interdependence on critical theory and (c) its social and professional organisation. I want to look at each of these in turn.

(a) *Critical thinking*

Over recent years, there has been a growth in academic critical thinking courses, initially as a supplement to more formal courses in logic. The skills associated with critical thinking, such as reflection, rational analysis and open-mindedness, are necessary to any academic endeavour and can be taught as methodological skills. They are now identified as a central aim of education in general. In schools in the UK, the 'AS' level in critical thinking has become increasingly popular (Fisher, 2001).

A cynical view may be that education in schools over recent years has left less room for individual thought. British universities are now looking at aptitude tests involving critical thinking skills to differentiate the best students at 'A' level. It may also be the case that the ideals of a liberal progressive education of the 1960s and 70s, which saw its aim as developing creative dissent rather than uncritical acceptance of orthodoxy, have now become seen as outmoded. At least critical thinking seems to be making a comeback, if only in its more regimented form as a method of learning that can be taught.

By critical thinking, I am not merely considering a technique that can be taught to improve problem solving. Maybe a better term is reflective practice, which involves a preparedness to think critically. The notion of reflection as a contribution to the improvement of practice has its origin in the work of John Dewey (1909). Doubt, perplexity and uncertainty lead to a search for possible explanations and solutions (Mamede & Schmidt, 2004). An attitude of openness means that the practitioner must tolerate the uncertainty and ambiguity required during reflection. 'Meta-reasoning' is the ability to think about one's own thinking processes and be prepared to critically assess one's own assumptions and beliefs.

Despite the development of guidelines and standards, which have been seen as being of increasing importance over recent years, professionals still need to use their judgement when undertaking their work. The National Institute for Clinical Excellence (NICE) agrees that guidelines may help healthcare professionals in their work, but that they cannot replace practitioners' knowledge and skills. Critical thinking is required to ensure that practice is open-minded, reflective and takes account of different perspectives. The route to clinical excellence is, in fact, through criticality, not reliance on managerial guidelines.

Critical thinking, then, is the art of taking charge of one's mind. If we can take charge of our own minds, the theory is that we can take charge of our lives; we can improve them, bringing them under our command and direction. Critical thinking involves getting into the habit of reflecting on our inherent and accustomed ways of thinking and leads to action in every dimension of our lives. Similarly, critical psychiatry wants to promote critical reflection on practice and research in psychiatry.

Critical thinking is not just having an impact in the field of psychiatry. For example, critical psychology (Fox & Prilleltensky, 1997) and critical social work (Adams et al, 2002) have been developed over recent years. The critical practitioner is someone who accepts uncertainty and attempts to deal with it creatively.

(b) Critical theory

More generally, critical psychiatry is based on critical theory. The term 'critical theory' is used quite loosely for a collection of theories critical of society and the human sciences (Thomas & Bracken, 2004). It applies to the theoretical basis of such fields as literature, philosophy, art, history, and the social sciences. Thus it can be applied to psychiatry as just one of these areas. Critical theorists include such people as Roland Barthes, Michel Foucault, Jacques Derrida, Julia Kristeva and Judith Butler, who do not necessarily fit easily into any one discipline. Michel Foucault (1967) has written particularly about psychiatry.

More specifically, the origin of the term 'critical theory' is in the approach of the group of German philosophers, sociologists and economists associated with the Frankfurt Institute for Social Research, and particularly the writings of Theodor Adorno, Max Horkheimer, Herbert Marcuse and Jürgen Habermas. Critical theory has distinguished itself through its critique of science as positivism. In other words, there is a tendency to believe that natural science is the only valid mode of knowledge and that progress continues to be made in uncovering facts through science. Psychiatry, for example, is said to have advanced over the years in its understanding of the mind and mental illness. It suits professional expectations to think that psychiatry has found the solution to the problem of mental illness. However, critical theory recognises that a rational basis of social existence has yet to be established, and, as such, is theoretically impossible.

Critical theory also seeks to explain how systems of collective beliefs legitimate various power structures. In relation to psychiatry, this can be applied to appreciating why people are so ready to adopt the biomedical model in psychiatry.

There could also be said to be a direct link between 'anti-psychiatry' and critical theory through Herbert Marcuse, who spoke at 'The dialectics of liberation' conference in 1967 organised by David Cooper, R.D. Laing and others (see chapter 2). Laing later said that the Frankfurt school of sociology never really appealed to him (Mullan, 1995: 217), but he did quote from *One dimensional man* (Marcuse, 1968) in his bestselling *The politics of experience* (Laing, 1967).

(c) Critical psychiatry as a social and professional activity

Besides being built on the notions of critical thinking and strengthened by critical theory, critical psychiatry has organised itself as a social and professional concern. I want to concentrate on the development of the Critical Psychiatry Network. To some extent at least, the definition of critical psychiatry must be understood by what the organisations that represent its principles actually do.

The Critical Psychiatry Network (www.criticalpsychiatry.co.uk) first met as the 'Bradford Group' in January 1999. It is a group of psychiatrists that forms a network to develop a critique of the contemporary psychiatric system. Similarly, the Critical Mental Health Forum (www.criticalmentalhealth.co.uk) has been meeting in London on a regular basis since January 2001. This is not a group made up of just one professional discipline. As well as professionals (ie. not only psychiatrists), the forum includes mental health service users, carers, academics and others who are critical of current theory and practice in mental health services.

The first meetings of the Critical Psychiatry Network (CPN) coincided with publication of the UK government's intention to undertake a root and branch review of the Mental Health Act 1983. This may be no coincidence as there are particular issues for critical psychiatry about the relation between coercion and mental health practice. Critical psychiatry does recognise the social role of psychiatry, and seeks a synthesis in the tension with psychiatry's therapeutic aims.

The initial phase of the review of the Mental Health Act involved a scoping exercise, undertaken by a small expert group chaired by Professor Genevra Richardson (Department of Health, 1999), to which CPN submitted evidence. CPN has also responded at each stage of the subsequent consultation process leading to the draft Mental Health Bill 2002. Its position statement in October 1999 made clear its opposition to compulsory treatment in the community, and preventive detention for people who are considered to have 'personality disorders'. A new response to the conflict between care and coercion was proposed that recognised the way values inform medical decisions. This perspective resists attempts to make psychiatry more coercive.

The Critical Psychiatry Network was an original member of the Mental Health Alliance (www.mentalhealthalliance.org.uk), a coalition of organisations that share common concerns about the government's proposals to reform the Mental Health Act. The core members have subsequently been joined by the Royal College of Psychiatrists, but initially CPN was the only group of psychiatrists that was part of the alliance. CPN's campaigning on the reform of the Mental Health Act has emphasised the importance of advance statements and rights to advocacy.

CPN has recently resigned from the Alliance, as it wishes to reserve its position about community treatment orders, on which the Alliance now seems prepared to compromise.

CPN is also currently campaigning against pharmaceutical company sponsorship of psychiatric conferences and educational activities. It believes that all organisations and conferences addressing psychiatric issues should provide full public disclosure of the amount of funding they receive from the psychiatric drug industry. A resolution to this effect was passed by the World Federation for Mental Health at its Membership Assembly held in Vancouver on 25 July 2001, so this stance is not a maverick position and does have general support. It is easy to blame the pharmaceutical industry for the over-prescription of psychotropic medication in society, but the medical profession itself needs to acknowledge its role. For example, much prescribing in bipolar disorder (manic-depressive illness) is outside licensed indications. It is clearly doctors who make the decision to prescribe in these circumstances, and they take the risk of prescribing 'off-licence'. There may be easy profits for the drug companies in this situation, but the medical profession should not allow itself to be exploited.

The Critical Psychiatry Network has a sceptical attitude to the use of psychotropic medication which has influenced contributions as a stakeholder to various guidelines produced by the National Institute for Clinical Excellence (NICE). For example, evidence provided to NICE by CPN on the efficacy of antidepressants has been ignored (Moncrieff & Kirsch, 2005). The scientific limits of the possibilities of randomised controlled trials should be more widely acknowledged, as should the general bias in the interpretation of the data. This does not mean that critical psychiatrists do not utilise medication in their practice – it is difficult to avoid its use in modern Western society – but they are equivocal about its merits. It is commonly assumed that the efficacy of psychotropic medication has been proven, but in fact it is more difficult than may be imagined to be sure that it is more effective than placebo. Critical psychiatry's challenge leads to the prescription of less medication. In fact, it is well-known that psychotropic medication is over-prescribed in ordinary clinical practice beyond that which can be justified from the evidence (Audit Commission, 1994). More could be done to intervene in this situation, possibly through the influence of NICE.

CPN has also organised and participated in various conferences, where papers have been presented which develop the notions on which critical psychiatry is based. Some of these papers have been published on the CPN website (www.criticalpsychiatry.co.uk), as have the other documents prepared by the group.

(ii) What are the key issues of critical psychiatry?

This book has examined the issues raised by critical psychiatry in some depth. It may be difficult to define what count as the key issues. Essentially critical psychiatry provides a paradigm for clinical practice (Double, 2005b). In other words, it incorporates a set of assumptions, concepts, values and practices that constitute a way of viewing psychiatry. In the real world, people do not always stick closely to the described model, and there may be variations of approach without being totally clear about what constitutes its essence.

Still, I think there is enough agreement about the nature of critical psychiatry to propose key principles in its foundation. I have adapted suggestions from an article by Thomas & Moncrieff (1999), the co-chairs of the Critical Psychiatry Network. Essentially these ideas amount to a critique of the biomedical model and its replacement by critical practice, which has an emphasis on the ethical and political dimensions of mental health problems. (Compare these notions with David Ingleby's understanding in chapter 4 of the main ingredients of the critical movement in mental health, also Ingleby, 2005). The Critical Psychiatry Network also produced a mission statement in March 2002 (www.criticalpsychiatry.co.uk/CPNmission.htm), which makes clear its underlying principles and describes its activities.

(a) A challenge to the dominance of clinical neurobiology in psychiatry (although this emphasis is not excluded)

The Critical Psychiatry Network is sceptical about the validity of the biomedical model of mental illness (see below for further discussion of the definition of the biomedical model). It disagrees with the emphasis placed on biological research and treatments and, as mentioned earlier, does not seek to justify psychiatric practice by postulating brain pathology as the basis for mental illness. Instead, it believes that the practice of psychiatry must recognise the primacy of social, cultural, economic and political contexts. These statements have been taken from the March 2002 mission statement.

An example of the bias of institutional psychiatry in favour of the biomedical model can be seen in a recent statement on the diagnosis and treatment of mental disorders from the American Psychiatric Association (APA) (2003). Despite the general suggestion that most psychiatrists now adopt a 'biopsychosocial' model of psychiatric illness, the APA maintains unequivocally that schizophrenia and other mental disorders are serious neurobiological disorders. The statement was issued in response to a hunger strike by six survivors of the psychiatric system (Mind Freedom, 2004). The challenge of the hunger strikers was that the APA should provide evidence to show that major mental illnesses are 'proven biological diseases of the brain' and that emotional distress results from 'chemical imbalances' in the brain.

The APA supported its contention by claiming that (i) research has shown reproducible abnormalities of brain structure and function (ii) evidence for a genetic component of mental disorders is compelling, and (iii) the mechanisms of action of effective medications have been elucidated. Each of these claims can be questioned (Double, 2004b). The APA no longer seems to be taking a pluralistic viewpoint on the biomedical aetiology of mental disorder, as it may have been expected to do in the past. It is misleading to say that most psychiatrists adopt the 'biopsychosocial' model when authoritative bodies speaking on behalf of psychiatry do not seem really to accept these foundations.

Psychiatric practice has become contingent on taking the step of faith of believing the biomedical hypothesis. Drug companies put advertisements in the medical press encouraging doctors to believe in their treatment. For the majority of conditions, however, research into genetics, brain chemistry, the physical environment and brain structure has not led to definite conclusions about physical causes (Kinderman & Cooke, 2000).

The problem with the claim that mental disorders are biological diseases is that it creates the reductionist tendency to treat people as brains that need their neuropathological lesions cured. Psychosocial factors in aetiology tend to be avoided. If biological and genetic factors determine psychopathology, the implication may be that personal and social efforts to improve one's state of mind may be pointless. This critique is not meant to imply that bodily factors can be ignored. Emotional problems clearly have physical effects. For example, stress can produce effects on the body and people are aware of the physiologic-al effects of adrenaline in the flight or fight response. In fact, the psychological origins of physical complaints are generally under-recognised.

Nor does it mean that critical psychiatry is unscientific in its approach. In fact, critical psychiatry argues that much of neurobiological research is insufficiently sceptical about its claims. After all, science should start from the 'null hypothesis'. The null hypothesis should only be rejected if the alternative hypothesis is sufficiently likely. Rarely does neurobiology have more than indicators to conclude that brain pathology is the cause of functional mental illness. Of course, not rejecting the null hypothesis does not necessarily mean it is true, but there is a need for more impartial research in the mental health field. Critical psychiatry shares the growing disquiet that corporate interests are compromising objective research.

(b) A strong ethical perspective on psychiatric knowledge and practice and the politicisation of mental health issues

Treating the biological abnormality and not the person, therefore, has ethical implications. It is often difficult to practise from a biomedical model in a way that really respects and engages with the patient's beliefs and preferences. What point is there in taking notice of the patient's view if you believe that the main objective is to rectify a neurochemical imbalance in someone's brain? The social model, on the other hand, recognises that the meaning of distress is culturally contingent, and so engaging with the person's belief systems and values is of paramount importance. This can only be achieved by listening carefully and respecting the person's beliefs.

One of critical psychiatry's most important tasks is the creation of a new dialogue between survivors, mental health service users and psychiatrists, a dialogue that recognises the value of different types of expertise. Psychiatrists are experts by profession, but service users are experts by experience. The best outcomes will only be achieved when these two types of expertise can work in alliance.

The notion that science can be theory free is too simple. Meanings as well as causes are essential to good psychiatric care (Fulford et al, 2003). Values ought to be just as much at the core of psychiatric explanatory models as scientific facts. Indeed, they are more explicit in psychiatry than they are in the rest of medicine. This is apparent in the nature of diagnostic criteria that are overtly evaluative in form (see chapter 5). It is to be expected in an area such as psychiatry, which is concerned with human emotions, desires, volition and beliefs.

Critical psychiatry also brings a political perspective on mental health issues. The biomedical model locates distress in the disordered function of the individual's mind/brain, which relegates social contexts to a secondary role. This is problematic because it completely overlooks the role of poverty and social exclusion in psychosis. Critical psychiatry is explicit about this social dimension.

The National Institute for Mental Health in England (NIMHE) has a programme of work to improve recognition of the importance of values, raise awareness of their impact and respect their diversity in mental health practice (Department of Health, 2004b). This development is welcome to temper the emphasis on scientific evidence in psychiatry. It has been based on the work of Bill Fulford (2004), who has enunciated the principles of Values-Based Medicine (VBM), seen as a counterpart to

Evidence-Based Medicine (EBM), an approach which has risen to prominence following the realisation that clinical decisions are not always necessarily based on the latest available evidence. This focus on values means that critical psychiatry must have a strong ethical foundation. The history of psychiatry demonstrates that the mentally ill have not always been well treated. Their rights and dignity need to be defended. For example, clear limits on the powers available under the Mental Health Act are required to ensure compassionate interventions.

(iii) How does critical psychiatry differ from mainstream psychiatry?

As mentioned above, at times, psychiatry has been more pluralistic than the current emphasis on the biomedical model would suggest. For example, Adolf Meyer's psychobiology focused on the patient as a person and was seen as an advance over the mechanistic views of the 19th century (see chapter 10). Psychoanalysis was more influential up to about 1970. In retrospect, the view that mental illnesses have primarily psychological causes could be regarded as a brief interlude in the history of psychiatry. By about 1970 the biological model of mental illness reasserted its dominance, as the power and attractiveness of psychoanalysis and Meyerian psychobiology declined.

This biomedical renaissance took place in the context of the increasing importance of psychopharmacology and attempts to make psychiatric diagnosis more reliable by the introduction of operational criteria, particularly in DSM-III. Psychiatry also had to withstand the critique of so-called 'anti-psychiatry'.

Counteracting 'anti-psychiatry' may have made orthodox psychiatry too defensive. Of course most clinicians are aware of the dangers of reducing people to their brains and avoid the worst excesses of the biomedical approach. Critical psychiatry argues that psychiatry needs to go further and clearly state it is not dependent on postulating brain pathology as the basis for mental illness. Even so-called 'eclectic' psychiatrists are rarely prepared to take this radical step.

The implications of this critical position affect diagnostic and therapeutic practice. An overemphasis on biomedical diagnosis is discouraged. Instead evaluation of the person in context is required. The dangers of 'labelling' are recognised. There is no doubt that psychiatric diagnosis is used inappropriately and in particular its use in the sense of biomedical disorder is unscientific (Boyle, 1990). There will inevitably be limitations in the application of psychiatric diagnosis, whatever way symptoms and signs are grouped and conceptualised. Critical psychiatry acknowledges this state of uncertainty. The concepts of mental illness may not need to be abandoned for this reason, but merely recognised for what they are – attempts to describe psychological states. They are therefore related to unobservables, and therefore not capable of description in the biomedical sense. Commonly, it is claimed that patients and relatives want a diagnosis, but giving one in biomedical terms may not add much to that meaning. Despite the difficulty of understanding the reasons for people's behaviour, critical psychiatry does try to engage with this issue with patients.

As far as treatment is concerned, critical psychiatry emphasises therapeutic practice in a general sense. The danger of mental health work is an overemphasis on custodial practice, and psychiatric services have to find a precarious balance alongside abuse and neglect. The maltreatment of patients in hospital was exposed in several scandals that gave an impetus to the dehospitalisation of patients (Martin 1984). Conversely, inquiries over recent years, particularly following homicides by psychiatric patients, have expressed concern about neglect of patients in the community (Peay 1996).

The 'sharp end' of psychiatry can still involve control and restraint, forced injections, ECT, close observations and seclusion. In this context, it is important not to lose sight of the person. Critical psychiatry emphasises the need for skills in communication in these difficult circumstances and the importance of creating a therapeutic environment.

For example, Diana Rose (2000) describes her treatment in a psychiatric ward.

> There was hardly any interaction between staff and patients. The interaction that did exist revolved around trouble. As long as there was something up, I got attention. When things were calmer and I was causing no trouble, I was ignored to the point of neglect. In the last few weeks, as I got ready for discharge, the boredom was crushing, even threatening to bring on another 'relapse'. The bureaucracy of the section 17 form did not help. Nurses communicated, as in other aspects, only to tell you what you could not do.

Her conclusion from this experience is that:

> The culture of psychiatry has to change so that people are not treated as 'cases' or instances of categories, but as people with hopes, fears and aspirations, which need to be dealt with on a human level.

There may be much to be re-learnt from the social therapy that developed with the unlocking of the psychiatric hospital doors in the 1950s and 60s (Clark, 1974). Modern psychiatry may be said to have reverted to the worst institutionalised behaviours of the asylums with its current climate of risk assessment and psychotropic drug management.

As also mentioned previously, critical psychiatry is sceptical about the efficacy of medication. Non-specific placebo effects can be powerful. Uncontrolled evaluation of the efficacy of treatment is undertaken by clinical trials and the acceptance and use of the double-blind method. Randomised controlled trials are commonly flawed in practice and the most rigorous trials are associated with less treatment benefit than poor quality trials. The double-blind method is not infallible because patients and doctors may be cued in to whether patients are taking active or placebo medication by a variety of means. These problems of unblinding may be minimised by trialists because there seems to be nothing that can be done to prevent it completely. Nonetheless, there should then be no pretence that unbiased evaluation of treatment is being carried out. Although the apparent specific effect of treatment may not be as great as the placebo effect itself, it may merely be the wishfulfilling amplification of non-specific effects.

The placebo effect may be relevant to problems in discontinuation of medication. People may form attachments to their medication more because of what it means to them than what it does. Any change threatens an equilibrium related to a complex set of meanings that their medication has acquired. These issues of reliance on medication should not be minimised, yet commonly compliance with treatment has been reinforced by emphasising that antidepressants, for example, are not addictive. Psychotropic medication is often prescribed in life crises reinforcing defensive mechanisms against overwhelming anxiety, and the power of the placebo effect should be recognised. Counteracting such placebo effects may not be easy when discontinuing medication.

Objectification of people by reducing them to abnormalities of their brains may not encourage an ethical relationship in treatment. Critical psychiatry is explicit that assessment and understanding of the person is required. Nonetheless, it still needs to be alert to the potential abuses of power of the 'healer' (Brody, 1992). The 'rescue fantasy' that only a particular therapist can cure a person's problems must constantly be kept in check by self-criticism and a true appreciation of the scientific evidence. Critical psychiatry is therefore well aware of the non-specific factors in psychiatric treatment. Treatment is about helping people muster resources to adapt and adjust to their problems.

The basis of modern biomedical psychiatry

I want to be clear about what I mean by the biomedical model. Criticism of the biomedical model is commonly deflected by suggesting that what is being attacked is not really held by most psychiatrists. In particular, many psychiatrists say that they are more eclectic in their approach to the factors in the aetiology of mental illness than merely relying on the biological.

It is true that some psychiatrists are more biomedical than others. The basic tenets may be held with varying degrees of conviction and awareness. Some clearly identify themselves as biological psychiatrists. Samuel Guze (1989), for example, says there is no other kind of psychiatry.

E. Fuller Torrey also, as another example, has no doubt that schizophrenia is a disease of the brain (Torrey & Kress, 2004). As far as he is concerned, scientific advances since 1975 have proven beyond reasonable doubt that schizophrenia is a disease of the brain. He notes that the 1959 *American handbook of psychiatry* (Arieti, 1959), by contrast, saw schizophrenia as 'a specific reaction to an extreme state of anxiety, originated in childhood and reactivated later in life by psychological factors'. This handbook described various psychoanalytic explanations of the origins of schizophrenia. According to Torrey, researchers stopped 'groping in the dark' with the publication of the first computerised axial tomography (CT) scan study of schizophrenia that revealed the enlarged cerebral ventricles of people diagnosed as schizophrenic compared to controls (Johnstone et al, 1976). He points to the evidence for neurological, neuropsychological, neurophysiological and cerebral metabolic abnormalities, as well as structural abnormalities. However, he does acknowledge that none of the potential abnormalities are specific for schizophrenia.

Torrey's belief in this evidence must explain the remarkable change in his understanding of the nature of mental illness. At the time of his book, *The death of psychiatry* (Torrey, 1974), Torrey agreed with Szasz's criticism of the concept of mental illness and was opposed, like Szasz, to involuntary psychiatric interventions and the insanity defence (Szasz, 2004b). He began his book with the dramatic statement, 'Psychiatry is dying', and by this he meant the medical model of human behaviour. Yet by the time he was writing *Surviving schizophrenia* (Torrey, 1983), he thought that schizophrenia is 'a brain disease, now definitely known to be such'. Biological psychiatry seems to have revived and Torrey is at the forefront of that resurrection. He is currently one of the most prominent advocates for forced psychiatric treatment in the United States. His change of heart, it has been suggested, may have been reinforced by the fortune donated by a wealthy couple with a mentally ill son to set up the Stanley Foundation (Carlson, 2001). Torrey became executive director of the Stanley Medical Research Institute.

My main reason for using Fuller Torrey as an illustration is the thoroughgoing nature of his biomedical perspective. He can see little reason for considering social and cultural factors in the aetiology of mental illness. He actually believes there has been a 'plague of brain dysfunction' that has occurred since the 18th century (Torrey & Miller, 2001). As far as he is concerned, asylums were not built for social or economic reasons, but merely to respond to the epidemic. The implication is that the mental hospitals should not have been emptied without ensuring adequate treatment to control the epidemic. His theory is that an infectious agent, or some other concomitant factor of industrialisation and urbanisation, causes schizophrenia. He is explicit that nonbiological factors play no part in aetiology, although they may influence the expression of symptoms. Schizophrenia and bipolar disorder are diseases of the brain, just as are Parkinson's disease and Alzheimer's disease.

This position may have the advantage of simplifying the relationship between mental illness and social and cultural factors. It also provides a logical consistency about the role of biological factors. The problem is to justify it conceptually and from the evidence. This book has thoroughly rehearsed the arguments against this biomedical hypothesis.

Other mainstream psychiatrists who adopt a biomedical perspective may be less convinced that the biological basis of mental illness has been proven, suggesting, for instance, that their perspective is eclectic, covering a broad range of different factors, including the biomedical. These authorities eschew a well-defined theoretical basis for practice. Neither constitutional nor environmental factors are said to predominate in aetiology. For example, Anthony Clare (1980) proposes that psychiatrists avoid adopting any one model. In his own words:

> Identifying the respective contributions of man, culture, and nature to the phenomenon of mental illness demands of psychiatrists, and of those who work alongside them, a willingness to avoid doctrinaire devotion to one or other of the ideologies competing for support and a determination to refrain from inflating the somewhat meagre items of genuine psychiatric knowledge into a programme of social reform and a political manifesto for the attainment of Utopia.
>
> Clare, 1980: 71

It is true that such eclecticism may avoid the worst excesses of reductionism. The problem is that it lacks a well-defined theoretical basis. It may introduce inconsistencies in that, for example, the psychosocial basis of minor mental disorders is recognised but severe mental illness is seen as primarily biological. This disparity may lead, for instance, to a combination of psychotherapy with medication in treatment without an appropriate integration in theory. Moreover, I want to argue that in effect eclecticism is still a variant of the biomedical model. A hint of this end result can be seen in Anthony Clare's summary of his chapter on 'The disease concept in psychiatry' in the textbook *The essentials of postgraduate psychiatry* (Murray et al 1997). Despite concluding that the pathogenesis of mental illness remains obscure, he goes on to suggest that:

> Nevertheless, there is a broad consensus within psychiatry, a consensus which has strengthened in recent years, to the effect that the advantages of the disease approach, the diagnostic process and the present rudimentary classification system outweigh the disadvantages.
>
> Clare, 1997b: 52

Although Clare had not really argued this case in the rest of the chapter, instead stating a more balanced view of the evidence, he seems to want to make this conclusion. Despite his well-meaning humanism, his position still seems determined by biologism.

To avoid misunderstanding, I want to be clear that I am not proposing a return to the psychoanalysis that dominated American psychiatry up to the 1960s. The current split between psychotherapy and biomedical psychiatry, loosely connected in mainstream eclectic psychiatry, does not really resolve the ideological issues in psychiatry. The view that psychotherapy is a treatment for 'psychologically based' disorders, while 'brain-based' disorders should be treated with medication, shows a dichotomised understanding of the relationship between mind and brain rather than an integrated approach (Luhrmann, 2000). An eclectic position seems to believe in the biomedical model as well as the benefits of psychotherapy, possibly in combined treatment with medication. By contrast, I want to suggest that critical psychiatry takes forward the Meyerian perspective that even psychotic disorders should be understood in psychosocial terms rather than reduced to brain abnormalities.

To illustrate this point, I have chosen a representative of modern social psychiatry. Julian Leff is well known for his contribution to work on the importance of expressed emotion in the families of people diagnosed as schizophrenic. He regards schizophrenia as still a 'puzzle', despite the advance in research over recent years (Leff, 1991). Even though identified with the social perspective in psychiatry, I want to show that Leff is not thoroughgoing in his opposition to the biomedical approach. If someone like Leff still upholds biologism, I think it reinforces my view that eclecticism is merely a weaker version of the biomedical model.

Leff (2001) in his book *The unbalanced mind* does not hide that he is more concerned to integrate a biological perspective with an understanding of the impact of the social environment, rather than challenge the importance of the biological basis of mental activity as such. Essentially he adopts a stress-diathesis model, rather than a more integrated Meyerian perspective, on the aetiology of mental illness. For example, he thinks manic-depressive illness is 'strongly determined by heredity' and that 'life events play an important role in setting the illness in motion, but it then develops a momentum of its own, perhaps driven by biochemical changes in the brain, and uninfluenced by environmental stress' (Leff 2001: 26). He makes much of the distinction between psychosis and neurosis and, for instance, believes in the value of lithium for controlling mood swings in manic-depressive illness. 'Experiences which are out of the ordinary', such as manic-depressive illness, are marked off from milder forms of depression, or 'an intensification of emotions that all humans feel', which as far as Leff is concerned do not respond to lithium. Leff does not demonstrate the same scepticism about psychotropic medication as does critical psychiatry (see chapter 7).

Leff (2001) also suggests that the World Health Organisation studies called the International Pilot Study of Schizophrenia (IPSS) and the Determinants of Outcome of Severe Mental Disorders (DOSMD) show that environmental factors play little part in the causation of schizophrenia. He does not seem to appreciate the strong bias in these studies towards discovering 'universals' in schizophrenia, and the way in which the results have been presented to minimise what are in fact still considerable differences in the presentation of schizophrenia in different countries (Kleinman, 1988).

Another example of Leff's uncritical attitude to biomedical beliefs is his acceptance of the value of antidepressants. He appears to welcome the fact that the Defeat Depression campaign, a public education campaign run jointly by the Royal Colleges of Psychiatrists and General Practitioners, led to an increase in the proportion of people endorsing antidepressants from 16 per cent in 1991 to 24 per cent in 1997 (Paykel et al, 1998). On the other hand, he laments the fact that the campaign did not change the public view that antidepressants are addictive, although the evidence is actually that there was a small significant drop in those with this belief from 78 to 74 per cent between 1991 and 1997 (Paykel et al,

1998). The issue of antidepressant discontinuation reactions, in fact, does seem to have been one in which the public could be said to have had a better appreciation than the medical profession of the extent to which antidepressants can be habit forming (Double, 1997). In contrast to advice from the Defeat Depression campaign just a few years earlier, guidelines from the National Institute for Clinical Excellence (2004) now clearly recommend that patients should be given a disclaimer about the risk of discontinuation/withdrawal symptoms when they first start anti-depressants. By encouraging patients to take antidepressants despite the risk of discontinuation reactions, Leff demonstrates his bias in favour of psychotropic medication. However to give Leff his due, most doctors were also taken in by the failure to recognise the nature of the problem.

Leff has more interest in the social perspective than most psychiatrists, for instance by studying the importance of urbanisation and race in the aetiology of mental disorder. However, the examples I have given show that he still adheres to an essentially biomedical model of mental illness, which leads to him being insufficiently critical of genetic theories of aetiology and the evidence base for psychotropic medication. My point is that modern psychiatry has real difficulties if even what is identified as social psychiatry does not really adopt a thoroughgoing psychosocial model, in the Meyerian sense, of mental illness.

Conclusion

I hope I have clarified what I mean by the biomedical model of mental illness and diffused the challenge that modern psychiatry is not really as biomedical as I suggest. In summary, simply stated, the biomedical model assumes underlying physical abnormalities are the cause of mental illness. Specifically, brain pathology explains mental illness. The rationale for this hypothesis is straightforward – as thought, emotion and behaviour have their origins in brain activity, abnormalities of thought, emotion and behaviour must also reside in the brain. I do not want to be misunderstood. I am not opposed to a materialistic understanding of the brain in the sense that the brain is seen as the origin of cognition, affect and behaviour. This logic is unassailable. The biological dimension can-not be denied. All thought, emotion and behaviour involve brain changes, and this is true for 'normal' experience as much as for abnormal experience such as mental illness. The problem is that the biomedical hypothesis takes a reductionist stance on the relationship between mind and brain. It does not sufficiently acknowledge that minds are enabled but not reducible to brains.

References

Abma, R. (1981) De katholieken en het psy-komplex. *Grafiet* 1: 156-97.

Adams, R., Dominelli, L. & Payne, M. (2002) *Critical practice in social work*. Basingstoke: Palgrave.

Adlam, D. & Rose, N. (1981) The politics of psychiatry. In: D. Adlam (ed.) *Politics and power. 4: Law, politics and justice*. London: Routledge & Kegan Paul.

Ainscow, M. & Tweddle, D.A. (1988) *Encouraging classroom success*. London: Fulton.

Alcock, P. & Harris, P. (1982) *Welfare, law and order: A critical introduction to law for social workers*. London: MacMillan.

Alweiss, L. (2000) (ed.) 'Special Edition on McDowell's *Mind and world*' for *The Journal of the British Society for Phenomenology*, 31: 3 Oct.

American Psychiatric Association (1952, 1968, 1980, 1987, 1994) *Diagnostic and statistical manual of mental disorders* (editions I-IV). Washington, D.C.: American Psychiatric Press.

American Psychiatric Association (1998) *Let's talk facts about childhood disorders*. American Psychiatric Association Pamphlet Series.

American Psychiatric Association (2003) *Statement on diagnosis and treatment of mental disorders*. Release no 03-39, September 25, 2003. www.psych.org/news_room/press_re leases/mentaldisorders0339.pdf.

Aries, P. (1998) From immodesty to innocence. In: H. Jenkins (ed.) *Children's culture reader*. New York: New York University Press.

Arieti, S. (1959) (ed.) *American handbook of psychiatry*. New York: Basic Books.

Armstrong, D. (1983) *The political anatomy of the body*. Cambridge: Cambridge University Press.

Aronowitz, S. & Giroux, H. (1991) *Post-modern education: Politics, culture and social criticism*. Minneapolis: University of Minnesota Press.

Audit Commission (1994) *A prescription for improvement – Towards more rational prescribing in general practice*. London: Audit Commission/HMSO.

Babyak, M., Blumenthal, J.A., Herman, S., et al (2000) Exercise treatment for major depression: maintenance of therapeutic benefit at 10 months. *Psychosomatic Medicine*, 62: 633-8.

Balbernie, R. (2001) Circuits and circumstances: The neurobiological consequences of early experiences and how they shape later behaviour. *Journal of Child Psychotherapy*, 27: 237-55.

Baldessarini, R.J., & Viguera, A.C. (1995) Neuroleptic withdrawal in schizophrenic patients. *Archives of General Psychiatry* 52: 189-92.

Baldwin, S. & Anderson, R. (2000) The cult of methylphenidate: Clinical update. *Critical Public Health*, 10: 81-6.

Baldwin, S. & Cooper, P. (2000) How should ADHD be treated? *The Psychologist* 13: 598-602

Barlow, G. & Hill, A. (1985) *Video violence and children*. London: Hodder and Stoughton.

Barnes, M. & Berke, J. (1971) *Mary Barnes. Two accounts of a journey through madness*. London: MacGibbon and Kee.

Barnes, M. & Bowl, R. (2001) *Taking over the asylum: Empowerment and mental health*. Basingstoke: Palgrave.

Barnes, M., Bowl, R. & Fisher, M. (1990) *Sectioned: Social services and the 1983 Mental Health Act*. London: Routledge.

Barton Evans III, F. (1996) *Harry Stack Sullivan. Interpersonal theory and psychotherapy.* London: Routledge.

Barton, R. (1959) *Institutional neurosis.* Bristol: Wright.

Basaglia, F. (1964) The destruction of the mental hospital as a place of institionalisation. www.triestesalutementale.it/inglese/allegati/FBASAGLIA1964.pdf (accessed 19 June 2004)

Basaglia, F. (1967) *L'istituzione negata.* Turin: Einaudi.

Basaglia, F.O. (1989) The psychiatric reform in Italy: Summing up and looking ahead. *International Journal of Social Psychiatry,* 35: 90-7.

Bateson, G., Jackson, D.D., Haley, J. & Weakland, J. (1956) Toward a theory of schizophrenia. *Behavioral Science,* 1: 251-64.

Baumeister, A.A. & Hawkins, M.F. (2001) Incoherence of neuroimaging studies in attention deficit/hyperactivity disorder. *Clinical Neuropharmacology,* 24: 2-10.

Becker, H.S. (1963) *Outsiders.* New York: Free Press.

Beer, M.D. (1995) Psychosis: From mental disorder to disease concept. *History of Psychiatry,* 6: 177-200.

Beer, M.D. (1996) The dichotomies: Psychosis/neurosis and functional/organic: A historical perspective. *History of Psychiatry,* 7: 231-55.

Beers, C.W. (1908) *The mind that found itself. An autobiography.* New York: Longmans, Green & Co.

Bentall, R. (2003) *Madness explained: Psychosis and human nature.* London: Allen Lane.

Beresford, P. (2005) Developing the theoretical basis for service user/survivor-led research and equal involvement in research. *Epidemiologia E Psichaitria Sociale,* 14: 4-9.

Beresford, P. & Croft. S. (1993) *Citizen involvement: A practical guide for change.* Basingstoke: Macmillan

Berke, J.H. (1977) *Butterfly man. Madness, degradation and redemption.* London: Hutchinson.

Biederman, J., Newcorn, J. & Sprich, S. (1991) Comorbidity of attention deficit disorder with conduct, depressive, anxiety and other disorders. *American Journal of Psychiatry,* 148: 564-77.

Blashfield, R.K. (1984) *The classification of psychopathology. Neo-Kraepelinian and quantitative approaches.* New York: Plenum

Bleuler, E. (1951) *Dementia praecox or the group of schizophrenias* (trans. J. Zinkin). London: Allen & Unwin.

Blumenthal, J.A., Babyak, M.A., Moore, K.A., et al (1999). Effects of exercise training on older patients with major depression. *Archives of Internal Medicine,* 159: 2349-56.

Bodenheimer, T. (2000) Uneasy alliance – clinical investigators and the pharmaceutical industry. *New England Journal of Medicine,* 342: 1539-44.

Bola, J.R. & Mosher L.R. (2003) treatment of acute psychosis without neuroleptics: two year outcomes from the Soteria project. *Journal of Nervous and Mental Disease,* 191: 219-29.

Bowden, C.L., Calabrese, J.R., McElroy, S.L., et al (2000). A randomized, placebo-controlled 12-month trial of divalproex and lithium in treatment of outpatients with bipolar I disorder. Divalproex Maintenance Study Group. *Archives of General Psychiatry,* 57: 481-9.

Bowden, C.L., Calabrese, J.R., Sachs, G., et al (2003). A placebo-controlled 18-month trial of lamotrigine and lithium maintenance treatment in recently manic or hypomanic patients with bipolar I disorder. *Archives of General Psychiatry,* 60: 392-400.

Bowlby, J. (1969) *Attachment and loss. Volume 1, Attachment.* London: Hogarth Press.

Bowlby, J. (1973) *Attachment and loss. Volume 2, Separation.* London: Hogarth Press.

Boyd, E.A. & Bero, L. (2000) Assessing faculty financial relationships with industry: a case study. *Journal of the American Medical Association,* 284: 2209-14.

Boyden, J. (1997) Childhood and the policy makers: A comparative perspective on the globalization of childhood. In: A. James & A. Prout (eds.) *Constructing and reconstructing childhood*. London: Falmer Press.

Boyers, R. & Orrill, R. (1972) (eds.) *Laing and anti-psychiatry*. Harmondsworth: Penguin.

Boyle, M. (1990, 2002a) *Schizophrenia: A scientific delusion?* (editions 1&2). London: Routledge.

Boyle, M. (1999). Diagnosis. In: C. Newnes, G. Holmes & C. Dunn (eds.) *This is madness: A critical look at psychiatry and the future of mental health services*. Ross-on-Wye: PCCS Books.

Boyle, M. (2002b) It's all done with smoke and mirrors. Or, how to create the illusion of a schizophrenic brain disease. *Clinical Psychology*, 12: 9-16.

Bracken, P. & Thomas, P. (2001) Post-psychiatry: a new direction for mental health. *British Medical Journal*, 322: 724-7.

Bracken, P. & Thomas, P. (2005) *Postpsychiatry: Mental health in a postmodern world*. Oxford: Oxford University Press.

Braslow, J. (1997) *Mental ills and bodily cures*. London: University of California Press.

Bray, S. & Preston-Shoot, M. (1995) *Empowerment and participation in social care*. Arnold.

Breger, L. (2000) *Freud*. New York: Wiley.

Breggin, P. (1985, 1991, 1993) *Toxic psychiatry*. New York: Fontana, 1985; New York: St. Martins Press, 1991; London: HarperCollins, 1993

Breggin, P. (1994) *Talking back to Prozac* New York: St. Martin's Paperbacks.

Breggin, P. (1999) Psycho-stimulants in the treatment of children diagnosed with ADHD: Part II. Adverse effects on brain and behavior. *Ethical Human Sciences and Services, 1*: 213-41.

Breggin, P. (2001) *Talking back to Ritalin: What doctors aren't telling you about stimulants for children* (revised edition). Cambridge, MA: Perseus Publishing.

Brewer, C. & Lait, J. (1978) *Can social work survive?* London: Temple Smith.

Brewer, S. (1999) Holistic doctor. *Chat magazine*, June.

Brinkgreve, Chr., Onland, J. & De Swaan, A. (1979) *De opkomst van het psycho-therapeutisch bedrijf (Sociologie van de psychotherapie, Vol. 1)*. Utrecht/Antwerpen: Aula/Het Spectrum.

British Medical Journal (2002) Theme issue 'Too much medicine?' *British Medical Journal*, 13 April, 324 (7342).

Brody, E.B. (1994) Psychiatric diagnosis in sociocultural context. *Journal of Nervous and Mental Disease*, 182: 253-6.

Brody, H. (1992) *The healer's power*. London: Yale University.

Brown, G. & Harris, T. (1978) *The social origin of depression*. London: Tavistock Publications.

Brown, P. (1990) The name game: Towards a sociology of diagnosis. *Journal of Mind and Behavior*, 11: 385-406.

Browne, E. & Finkelhor, D. (1986) The impact of child sexual abuse: A review of the research. *Psychological Bulletin*, 99: 66-77.

Browne, I. (1999) *Sunday Business Post*, 11 July.

Bulmer, M. (1987) *The social base of community care*. London: Heinmann.

Burns, C.L.C. (1954) A forgotten psychiatrist – Baron Ernst von Feuchtersleben, M.D., 1833. *Proceedings of the Royal Society of Medicine*, 47: 190-4.

Calvert, K. (1992) *Children in the house: The material culture of early childhood, 1600-1900*. Boston: Northeastern University Press.

Campbell, J. (1998) Unified mental health teams: the Northern Ireland case. *Conference on collaborative mental health approaches, Anglia Polytechnic University and the Sainsbury Centre*, February.

Capra, F. (1997) *The web of life: A new synthesis of mind and matter*. London: Flamingo.

Carlowe, J. (2002) Back to the beginning. *The Observer Magazine*, 20 January, p. 53.

Carlson, P. (2001) Thinking outside the box: E. Fuller Torrey has brains. *The Washington Post*, Monday 9 April.

Caron, C. & Rutter, M. (1991) Comorbidity in child psychopathology: concepts, issues and research strategies. *Journal of Child Psychology and Psychiatry*, 32: 1063-80.

Carpenter, W.T. Jr., Mcglashan, T.H. & Strauss, J.S. (1977) The treatment of acute schizophrenia without drugs: an investigation of current assumptions. *American Journal of Psychiatry*, 134: 14-20.

Castellanos, F.X., Lee, P.P., Sharp, W., et al (2002) Developmental trajectories of brain volume abnormalities in children and adolescents with attention-deficit/hyperactivity disorder. *Journal of the American Medical Association*, 288: 1740–8.

Castillo, H. (2003) *Personality disorder: Temperament or truama?* London: Jessica Kingsley, Forensic Focus 23.

Charles, L. & Schain, R. (1981) A four year follow up study of the effects of methylphenidate on the behaviour and academic achievement of hyperactive children. *Journal of Abnormal Child Psychology*, 9: 495-505.

Chess, S. & Thomas, A. (1996) *Temperament theory and practice*. New York: Brunner Mazel.

Chilvers, C., Dewey, M., Fielding, K., et al (2001) Antidepressant drugs and generic counselling for treatment of major depression in primary care: randomised trial with patient preference arms. *British Medical Journal*, 322: 772-5.

Christie, D., Lieper, A.D., Chessells, J.M. & Vergha-Khadem, F. (1995) Intellectual performance after presymptomatic cranial radiotherapy for leukaemia: effects of age and sex. *Archives of Disease in Childhood*, 73: 136-40.

Ciompi, L., Kupper, Z., Aebi, E., et al (1993) Das pilotprojekt 'Soteria Berne' zur behandlung akut schizophrener. *Nervenarzt*, 64: 440-50.

Clare, A. (1980) *Psychiatry in dissent* (second edition). London: Routledge.

Clare, A. (1997a) In: B. Mullan (ed.) *R.D. Laing: Creative destroyer*. London: Cassell

Clare, A. (1997b) The disease concept in psychiatry. In: R. Murray, P. Hill & P. McGuffin (eds.) *The essentials of postgraduate psychiatry*. Cambridge: Cambridge University Press.

Clark, D.H. (1974) *Social therapy in psychiatry*. Harmondsworth: Penguin.

Colbert, T. (2001a) *Rape of the soul: How the chemical imbalance model of modern psychiatry has failed its patient*. California: Kevco Publishing.

Colbert, T. (2001b) *Blaming our genes: Why mental illness can't be inherited*. California: Kevco Publishing.

Collier, A. (1977) *R.D. Laing: The philosophy and politics of psychotherapy*. Hassocks: Harvester Press.

Conrad, P. (1980) On the medicalisation of deviance and social control. In: D. Ingleby (ed.) *Critical psychiatry: The politics of mental health*. New York: Pantheon, pp. 102-19.

Cooper, D. (1967) *Psychiatry and anti-psychiatry*. London: Tavistock.

Cooper, D. (1968) (ed.) *The dialectics of liberation*. Harmondsworth: Penguin.

Cooper, D. (1971) *The death of the family*. Harmondsworth: Penguin.

Cooper, D. (1974) *The grammar of living*. London: Allen Lane.

Cooper, D. (1980) *The language of madness*. Harmondsworth: Pelican.

Cooper, R. (1994) (with S. Gans, J.M. Heaton, H. Oakley & P. Zeal) Beginnings. In: R. Cooper, J. Friedman, S. Gans, J.M. Heaton, C. Oakley, H. Oakley & P. Zeal *Thresholds between philosophy and psychoanalysis*. London: Free Association Books.

Cunningham, H. (1995) *Children and childhood in western society since 1500*. London: Longman.

Daniels, H., Hey, V., Leonard, D. & Smith, M. (1998) Difference, difficulty and equity: Gender race and SEN. *Management in Education*, 12: 5-8.

Davis, K. (1986) The process of problem (re)formulation in psychotherapy. *Sociology of Health & Illness*, 8: 44-74.

Deleuze, G. (1983) *Nietzsche and philosophy* (trans. H. Tomlinson). London: Athlone Press.

Deleuze, G. & Guattari, F. (1977) *Anti-oedipus: Capitalism and schizophrenia.* New York: Viking.

Department of Health (1998a) Frank Dobson outlines third way for mental health (press release reference no 98/311). www.dh.gov.uk/PublicationsAndStatistics/PressReleases/PressReleasesNotices/fs/en?CONTENT_ID=4024509&chk=G4JMRG

Department of Health (1998b) *Modernising mental health services.* London: Department of Health.

Department of Health (1999) *Review of the Mental Health Act 1983: Report of the expert committee.* London: Stationery Office.

Department of Health (2002) *Prescription cost analysis 2001.* London: Stationery Office.

Department of Health (2004a) *The national service framework for mental health – Five years on.* London: Stationery Office

Department of Health (2004b) *The ten essential shared capabilities.* London: Stationery Office.

Dewey, J. (1909) *How we think.* London: Heath.

Diggins, M. (2000) Innovation as a way of professional life – the Building Bridges Project for parent-users of mental health services and their children. In: S. Ramon (ed.) *A stakeholder's approach to innovation in mental health services: A reader for the 21st century.* Brighton: Pavilion Publishing, pp. 75-91.

Double, D.B. (1997) Prescribing antidepressants in general practice. People may become psychologically dependent on antidepressants. *British Medical Journal,* 314: 826.

Double, D.B. (2002) The limits of psychiatry. *British Medical Journal,* 324: 900-4.

Double, D.B. (2004a) Suspension of doctors: Medical suspensions may have ideological nature. *British Medical Journal,* 328: 709-10.

Double, D.B. (2004b) Biomedical bias of the American Psychiatric Association. *Ethical Human Psychology and Psychiatry,* 6: 153-9.

Double, D.B. (2005a) Beyond biomedical models: A perspective from critical psychiatry. In: J. Tew (ed.) *Social perspectives in mental health: Developing social models to understand and work with mental distress.* London: Jessica Kingsley, pp. 53-70.

Double, D.B. (2005b) Paradigm shift in psychiatry. In: S. Ramon & J. Williams (eds.) *Mental health at the crossroads.* Aldershot: Ashgate.

Dowrick, C., Dunn, G., Ayuso-Mateos, J.L., et al (2000) Problem solving treatment and group psychoeducation for depression: Multicentre randomised controlled trial. *British Medical Journal,* 321: 1450-4.

Duggan, M. (2002a) (with Cooper, A. & Foster, J.) *Modernising the social model in mental health: A discussion paper.* London: Social Perspectives Network for Modern Mental Health/TOPSS England www.spn.org.uk/fileadmin/SPN_uploads/Documents/spn_paper_1_RP.pdf.

Duggan, M. (2002b) Policy prescriptions. *Community Care,* 14-20 February, pp. 38-9.

Editor (1915) Editorial. *Journal of Mental Science,* 61: 501-2.

Eisenberg, L. (1986) Mindlessness and brainlessness in psychiatry. *British Journal of Psychiatry,* 148: 497-508.

Eisenberg, L. (1995) The social construction of the human brain. *American Journal of Psychiatry,* 152: 1563-75.

El-Hai, J. (2005) *The lobotomist. A maverick medical genius and his tragic quest to rid the world of mental illness.* Hoboken, N.J.: Wiley.

Engel, G.L. (1977) The need for a new medical model: a challenge for biomedicine. *Science,* 196: 129-36.

Esterson, A. (1972) *The leaves of spring.* Harmondsworth: Pelican.

Esterson, A. (1976) Anti-psychiatry (letter). *The New Review,* 3: 70-1.

Esterson, A., Cooper, D.G. & Laing, R.D. (1965) Results of family orientated schizophrenics with hospitalised schizophrenics. *British Medical Journal*, 5476: 1462-5.

Ewins, D. (1974) Unpublished MA thesis, University of Sheffield. Quoted in Unsworth, 1987: 258.

Fadden, G. (1998) Research update: psychosocial interventions. *Journal of Family Therapy*, 20: 293-309.

Fanon, F. (1967) *The wretched of the earth*. Harmondsworth: Penguin.

Farrell, B.A. (1979) Mental illness: a conceptual analysis. *Psychological Medicine*, 9: 21-35.

Feighner, J.P., Robins, E., Guze, S.B., et al (1972) Diagnostic criteria for use in psychiatric research. *Archives of General Psychiatry*, 26: 57-63.

Fergusson, D.M. & Horwood, L.J. (1993) The structure, stability and correlations of the trait components of conduct disorder, attention deficit disorder and anxiety withdrawal reports. *Journal of Child Psychology and Psychiatry*, 34: 749-66.

Fernando, S. (1991) *Mental health, race and culture*. London: Macmillan.

Feuchtersleben, E. von (1976) *The principles of medical psychology* (reprint edition). New York: Arno Press.

Fisher, A. (2001) *Critical thinking: An introduction*. Cambridge: University Press .

Fisher, S. & Greenberg, R.P. (1989) *The limits of biological treatments for psychological distress*. Hillsdale, N.J.: Erlbaum.

Fisher, S. & Greenberg, R.P. (1997) *From placebo to panacea*. New York: John Wiley & Sons.

Fisher, S.L., Francks, C., McCracken, J.T., et al (2002). A genome-wide scan for loci involved in attention deficit/hyperactivity disorder (ADHD). *American Journal of Human Genetics*, 70: 1183-96.

Fodor, J.A. (1983) *The modularity of mind*. Cambridge, MA: MIT Press.

Fombonne, E., Wostear, G., Cooper, V., et al (2001) The Maudsley long-term follow-up of child and adolescent depression 1. Psychiatric outcomes in adulthood. *British Journal of Psychiatry*, 179: 210-17.

Forti, L. (2002) Then and now. In: J.H. Berke, M. Fagan, G. Mak-Pearce & S. Pierides-Mueller (eds.) *Beyond madness: PsychoSocial interventions in psychosis*. London: Jessica Kingsley.

Foster, N. (2005) Control, citizenship and 'risk' in mental health: perspectives from UK, USA and Australia. In: S. Ramon & J. Williams (eds.) *Mental health at the crossroads: The promise of the psychosocial approach*. Aldershot: Ashgate, pp. 30-42.

Foucault, M. (1967) *Madness and civilization: A history of insanity in the Age of Reason* (trans. R. Howard). London: Tavistock.

Foucault, M. (1981) *The history of sexuality*. Harmondsworth: Penguin.

Foucault, M. (1988) *The final Foucault* (edited by J. Bernauer & D. Rasmussen). Cambridge MA: MIT Press.

Foucault, M. (1991) *Governmentality*. In: G. Burchell, C. Gordon & P. Miller (eds.) *The Foucault effect: Studies in governmentality*. Chicago: University of Chicago Press.

Foucault, M. (1993) *Dream and existence* (edited by K. Hoeller). New Jersey: Humanities Press.

Foucault, M. (2001) *Fearless speech* (Edited by J. Pearson). Los Angeles: Semiotext(e).

Foucault, M. (2003) *Abnormal* (trans. G. Burchell). London: Verso.

Foudraine, J (1974). *Not made of wood: A psychiatrist discovers his own profession* (trans. from the Dutch by Hubert H. Hoskins). London: Quartet Books.

Foudraine, J. (2001) On the power of medical maya: An update of 'Not made of wood'. Keynote address at Critical Psychiatry Network conference, Sheffield, 27 April 2001 (available at www.criticalpsychiatry.co.uk/Foudraine.htm).

Fox, D. & Prilleltensky, I. (1997) (eds.) *Critical psychology: An introduction*. London: Sage

Fox, N.A., Rubin, K.H., Calkins, S.D., et al (1995) Frontal activation asymmetry and social competence at four years of age. *Child Development*, 66: 1770-84.

Free Association Books (2004) Book information about *Critical Psychiatry* www. fabooks.com/book.php?id=383 (accessed 9 April 2004).

Freeman, W. & Watts, J.W. (1950) *Psychosurgery in the treatment of mental disorders and intractable pain.* Springfield, Illinois: Thomas.

Freud, S. (1910) The origin and development of psychoanalysis. *American Journal of Psychology*, 21: 181-218.

Freud, S. (1911) *Formulations on the two principles of mental functioning.* Standard Edition of the Complete Psychological Works of Sigmund Freud 12: 213.

Fulford, K.W.M. (1994) Closet logics: hidden conceptual elements in the DSM and ICD classification of mental disorders. In: J.Z. Sadler, O.P. Wiggins, & M.A. Schwartz (eds.) *Philosophical perspectives on psychiatric diagnostic classification.* Baltimore: Johns Hopkins University Press. pp. 211-13.

Fulford, K.W.M. (2004) Ten principles of values-based medicine. In: J. Radden (ed.) *The philosophy of psychiatry: A companion.* New York: Oxford University Press, pp. 205-34

Fulford, K.W.M. (Bill), Morris, K., Sadler, J. & Stanghellini, G. (2003) *Nature and narrative: An introduction to the new philosophy of psychiatry.* Oxford: Oxford Univerity Press.

Furedi, F. (2004) *Therapy culture.* London: Routledge.

Gadow, K.D. (1983) Effects of stimulant drugs on academic performances in hyperactivity and learning disabled children. *Journal of Learning Disabilities*, 16: 290-9.

Gaines, A. (1992) *Ethnopsychiatry: The cultural construction of professional and folk psychiatries.* Albany: State University of New York Press.

Galvin, S.W. & McCarthy, S. (1994) Multidisciplinary community teams: Clinging to the wreckage. *Journal of Mental Health*, 3: 167-74.

Gans, S. & Redler, L. (2001) (in conversation with B. Mullan) *Just listening.* Philadelphia: Xlibris Corporation.

Garber, S.W., Garber, M.D. & Spizman, R.F. (1996) *Beyond Ritalin.* New York: Harper Perennial.

Gelder, M. (1991) Adolf Meyer and his influence on British psychiatry. In: G. Berrios & H. Freeman (eds.) *150 years of British psychiatry, 1841-1991.* London: The Royal College of Psychiatrists.

Gijswijt-Hofstra, M. & Porter, R. (1998) (eds.) *Cultures of psychiatry and mental health care in post-war Britain and Netherlands.* Amsterdam: Clio Medica.

Glouberman, S. (2001) *Towards a new perspective on health policy.* Canadian Policy Research Network study no. W/03.

Goffman, E. (1961) *Asylums. Essays on the social situation of mental patients and other inmates.* Harmondsworth: Penguin.

Goffman, E. (1969) *The presentation of self in everyday life.* London: Allen Lane

Goodman, R. (1997) An over extended remit? *British Medical Journal*, 314: 813-14.

Goodwin S. (1997) *Comparative mental health policy: From institutional to community care.* London: Sage.

Gove, W. (1980) (ed.) *The labelling of deviance.* London: Sage.

Green, M., Wong, M., Atkins, D., et al (1999). *Diagnosis of attention deficit hyperactivity disorder.* Rockville, MA: Agency for Healthcare Policy and Research.

Greenhalgh, T. & Hurwitz, B. (1998) (eds.) *Narrative based medicine.* London: BMJ Books.

Grob, G.N. (1963) Adolf Meyer on American psychiatry in 1895. *American Journal of Psychiatry*, 119: 1135-42.

Grob, G.N. (1983) *The inner world of American psychiatry 1890-1940.* New Brunswick: Rutgers University Press.

Guze, S.B. (1989) Biological psychiatry: Is there any other kind? *Psychological Medicine*, 19: 315-23.

Habermas, J. (1987) *The theory of communicative action, Vol II: System and lifeworld* (original German edition, 1981). Cambridge: Polity Press.

Halperin, D. (1995) *Saint Foucault: Towards a gay hagiography*. Oxford: Oxford University Press.

Harper, P. & Clarke, A. (1997) *Genetics, society and clinical practice*. London: Bios Scientific Publications.

Harrington, R. (1994) Affective disorders. In: M. Rutter, E. Taylor & L. Hersov (eds.) *Child and adolescent psychiatry. Modern approaches* (third edition). Oxford: Blackwell Scientific.

Harrington, R., Fudge, H., Rutter, M., et al (1993) Child and adult depression: a test of continuities with data from a family study. *British Journal of Psychiatry*, 162: 627-33.

Harrop, C. & Trower, P. (2003) *Why does schizophrenia develop at late adolescence? A cognitive-developmental approach to psychosis*. Chichester: Wiley.

Healy, D. (1997) *The antidepressant era*. Cambridge, MA: Harvard University Press.

Healy, D. (1998) Gloomy days and sunshine pills. *Openmind*, 90: 8-9.

Heaton, J.M. (2000) *Wittgenstein and psychoanalysis*. Cambridge: Icon Books.

Hendrick, H. (1997) Constructions and reconstruction's of British childhood: An interpretive survey, 1800 to the present. In: A. James & A. Prout (eds.) *Constructing and reconstructing childhood*. London: Falmer Press.

Hennelly, R. (1990) Mental health resource centres. In: S. Ramon (ed.) *Psychiatry in transition: British and Italian experiences*. London: Pluto Press.

Henry, J. (1963) *Culture against man*. New York: Vintage.

Hetchman, L., Weis, G. & Perlman, T. (1984) Young adult outcome of hyperactive children who received long term stimulant medication. *Journal of the American Academy of Child and Adolescent Psychiatry*, 23: 261-9.

Hey, V., Leonard, D., Daniels, H. & Smith, M. (1998) Boys' underachievement, special needs practices and questions of equity. In: D. Epstein, J. Elwood, V. Hey & J. Maw (eds.) *Failing boys? Issues in gender and underachievement*. Buckingham: Open University Press.

Heyman, R. (1994) Methylphenidate (Ritalin): Newest drug of abuse in schools. *Ohio Pediatrics*, Spring: 17-18.

Hill, D. (1993) Psychiatry's lost cause, *Openmind*, 61: 16-17.

Hill, P. (1997) Child and adolescent psychiatry. In: R. Murray, P. Hill & P. McGuffin (eds.) *The essentials of postgraduate psychiatry* (third edition). Cambridge: Cambridge University Press.

Houston, M. (2001) Irish Times medical correspondent, *The Irish Times*, 17 December 2001.

Huxley P., Evans S., Gately C. & Webber M. (2003) *Workload and working patterns among mental health social workers: An investigation into occupational pressures*. London: Social Work Social Care Section, Health Services Research Department.

Huxley, P. Evans, S., Webber M. & Gately, C. (2004) *Survey of mental health social workers in England and Wales*. London: Social Care Workforce Research Unit.

Hynd, G.W. & Hooper, S.R. (1995) *Neurological basis of childhood psychopathology*. London: Sage Publications.

Hypericum Depression Trial Study Group (2002) Effect of hypericum perforatum (St John's Wort) in major depressive disorder: A randomized controlled trial. *Journal of the American Medical Association*, 287: 1807-14.

Ingleby, D. (1980a, 1981, 2004) (ed.) *Critical psychiatry: The politics of mental health*. First impression, New York: Pantheon, 1980; Harmondsworth: Penguin, 1981. Second impression, London: Free Association Books, 2004.

Ingleby, D. (1980b) Understanding 'mental illness'. In: D. Ingleby (ed.) *Critical psychiatry: The politics of mental health*, (see above), pp. 23-71

Ingleby, D. (1982) The social construction of mental illness. In: A. Treacher & P. Wright (eds.) *The problem of medical knowledge: Examining the social construction of medicine*. Edinburgh: Edinburgh University Press. pp. 123-43.

Ingleby, D. (1983) Mental health and social order. In: S. Cohen & A. Scull (eds.) *Social control and the state*. London: Martin Robertson, pp. 141-88.

Ingleby, D. (1985) Professionals as socialisers: The 'psy complex'. In: A. Scull & S. Spitzer (eds.) *Research in law, deviance and social control 7*. New York: Jai Press, pp. 79-109.

Ingleby, D. (1998) A view from the North Sea. In: M. Gijswijt-Hofstra & R. Porter (eds.) *Cultures of psychiatry*. Amsterdam: Rodopi.

Ingleby, D. (2005) The origins of critical psychiatry. Lecture given at annual meeting of Royal College of Psychiatrists, Edinburgh, 22 June 2005 (available at www.critical psychiatry.co.uk/Edinburgh1.htm).

Jacyna, L.S. (1982) Somatic theories of mind and the interests of medicine in Britain 1850-1879. *Medical History*, 16: 233-58.

James, W. (1907) What pragmatism means. Lecture 2. In: *Pragmatism: A new name for some old ways of thinking*. New York: Longman Green and Co, pp. 17-32. http://spartan.ac.brocku.ca/~lward/James/James_1907/James_1907_02.html (accessed 21 April 2005).

Jaspers, K. (1963). *General psychopathology* (trans J. Hoenig & M.W. Hamilton). Manchester: Manchester University Press.

Jenhs, C. (1996) *Childhood*. London: Routledge.

Jenkins, H. (1998) Introduction: Childhood innocence and other modern myths. In: H. Jenkins (ed.) *The children's culture reader*. New York: New York University Press.

Jenkins, R. (1995) quoted in L. Boley, Draining the gene pool, *Openmind*, 74: 16-17.

Johnson, F.N. (1984) *The history of lithium therapy*. London: Macmillan.

Johnson, T. (1995) Governmentality and the institutionalisation of expertise. In: T. Johnson, G. Larkin & M. Saks (eds.) *Health professions and the state in Europe*. London: Routledge.

Johnstone, E.C., Crow, T.J., Frith, C.D., et al (1976) Cerebral ventricular size and cognitive impairment in schizophrenia. *Lancet*, ii: 924-6.

Johnstone, E.C., Macmillan, J.F., Frith, C.D., et al (1990) Further investigation of outcome following first episode schizophrenic episodes. *British Journal of Psychiatry*, 158: 713-4.

Johnstone, E.C., Freeman, C.P.L. & Zeally, A.K. (1998) *Companion to psychiatric studies* (sixth edition). Edinburgh: Churchill Livingstone.

Johnstone, L. (2000) *Users and abusers of psychiatry: A critical look at psychiatric practice* (second edition). London: Routledge.

Jones, C. (1998) Raising the anti: Jan Foudraine, Ronald Laing and anti-psychiatry. In: M. Gijswijt-Hofstra & R. Porter (eds.) *Cultures of psychiatry*. Amsterdam: Editions Rodopi, pp. 283-94.

Jones, M. (1952) *Social psychiatry*. London: Tavistock.

Jones-Edwards, G (1993) An eye-opener. *Openmind*, September/October: 9-10 & 19.

Joseph. J. (2004) *The gene illusion: Genetic research in psychiatry and psychology under the microscope*. Ross-on-Wye: PCCS Books.

Joughin, C. & Zwi, M. (1999). *Focus on the use of stimulants in children with attention deficit hyperactivity disorder. Primary evidence-base briefing No.1*. London: Royal College of Psychiatrists Research Unit.

Jureidini, J., Doecke, C., Mansfield, P.R., et al (2004a) Efficacy and safety of anti-depressants for children and adolescents. *British Medical Journal*, 328: 879-83.

Jureidini, J., Tonkin, A. & Mansfield, P. (2004b) TADS study raises concerns. *British Medical Journal*, *329*: 1343-4.

Kafka, F. (1991) *The blue octavo notebooks*. (ed. Max Brod). Cambridge, MA: Exact Change.

Kant, I. (1997) *Critique of practical reason* (trans. M. Gregor). Cambridge: Cambridge University Press.

Kant, I. (1998) *Critique of pure reason* (trans. P. Guyer & A.W. Wood). Cambridge: University Press.

Keller, M.B., Kocsis, J.H., Thase, M.E., et al (1998) Maintenance phase efficacy of sertraline for chronic depression. *Journal of the American Medical Association*, 280: 1665-72.

Kidd, K. (2000) quoted in E. Goode, Reading the book of life, *New York Times*, June 27.

Kiesler, D.J. (1999) *Beyond the disease model of mental disorders*. Praeger: Westport, Connecticut.

Kincheloe, J. (1998) The new childhood; Home alone as a way of life. In: H. Jenkins (ed.) *Children's culture reader*. New York: New York University Press.

Kinderman, P. & Cooke, A. (2000) (eds.) *Recent advances in understanding mental illness and psychotic experience. A report of the British Psychological Society Division of Clinical Psychology*. Leicester: British Psychological Society.

Kirk, S. & Kutchins, H. (1994) The myth of the reliability of DSM. *Journal of Mind and Behaviour*, 15: 71-86.

Kirkby, K.C. (1992) Proving the somaticist position: J.B. Friedreich on the nature and seat of mental disease. *History of Psychiatry*, 3: 237-51.

Kirsch, I., Moore, T.J., Scoboria, A. & Nicholls, S.S. (2002) The emperor's new drugs: an analysis of antidepressant medication data submitted to the U.S. Food and Drug Administration. *Prevention & Treatment*, 5, Article 23.   www.journals.apa.org/prevention/volume5/pre0050023a.html

Kirsner, D. (2000) *Unfree associations*. London: Process Press.

Klein, R.G. & Mannuzza, S. (1991) Long-term outcome of hyperactive children: A review. *Journal of the American Academy of Child and Adolescent Psychiatry*, 30: 383-7.

Kleinman, A. (1988) *Rethinking psychiatry. From cultural cateogory to personal experience*. New York: Free Press.

Klerman, G.L. (1978) The evolution of a scientific nosology. In: J.C. Shershow (ed.) *Schizophrenia: Science and Practice*. Cambridge, MA: Harvard University Press.

Knight, C. (1978) *Neighbourhood support groups*. London: Family Welfare Association..

Kovel, J. (1980) The American mental health industry. In: D. Ingleby (ed.) *Critical psychiatry: Tthe politics of mental health*. London: Penguin.

Kraepelin, E. (1921) *Manic-depressive insanity and paranoia*. Edinburgh: Livingstone.

Kuipers, L., Leff, J. & Lam, D. (1992) *Family work for schizophrenia: A practical guide*. London: Gaskell.

Kutchins, H. & Kirk, S. (1999) *Making us crazy. DSM: The psychiatric bible and the creation of mental disorders*. London: Constable.

Laing, R.D. (1960) *The divided self*. London: Tavistock.

Laing, R.D. (1961) *Self and others*. London: Tavistock Publications.

Laing, R.D. (1967) *The politics of experience & The bird of paradise*. Harmondsworth: Penguin.

Laing, R.D. (1970) *Knots*. London: Tavistock.

Laing, R.D. (1971) *The politics of the family and other essays*. London: Tavistock.

Laing, R.D. (1972) Metanoia: Some experiences at Kingsley Hall, London. In: H.M. Ruitenbeek (ed.) *Going crazy. The radical therapy of R.D. Laing and others*. New York: Bantam.

Laing, R.D. (1976) *The facts of life*. London: Allen Lane.

Laing, R.D. (1977) *Do you love me?* London: Allen Lane.

Laing, R.D. (1978) *Conversations with children*. London: Allen Lane.

Laing, R.D. (1979a) *Sonnets*. London: Joseph.

Laing, R.D. (1979b) Round the bend. Review of *The theology of medicine, The myth of psychotherapy & Schizophrenia* by T.S. Szasz. *New Statesman*, July 20.

Laing, R.D. (1982) *The voice of experience*. London: Allen Lane.

Laing, R.D. (1985) *Wisdom, madness and folly*. London: Macmillan.

Laing, R.D. (1987) Laing's understanding of interpersonal experience. In: R.L. Gregory (ed.) (assisted by O.L. Zangwill) *The Oxford companion to the mind*. Oxford: Oxford Univeristy Press.

Laing, R.D. & Cooper D.G. (1964) *Reason and violence*. London: Tavistock.

Laing, R.D. & Esterson, A. (1964) *Sanity, madness and the family*. Volume 1. *Families of schizophrenics*. London: Tavistock.

Lambert, N.M. & Hartsough, C.S. (1998) Prospective study of tobacco smoking and substance dependence among samples of ADHD and non-ADHD participants. *Journal of Learning Disabilities*, 31: 533-44.

Laor, N. (1982) Szasz, Feuchtersleben, and the history of psychiatry. *Psychiatry*, 45: 316-24.

LeFever, G.B., Dawson, K.V. & Morrow, A.D. (1999) The extent of drug therapy for attention deficit hyperactivity disorder among children in public schools. *American Journal of Public Health*, 89: 1359-64.

Leff, J. (1991) Schizophrenia in the melting pot. *Nature*, 353: 693-4.

Leff, J. (2001) *The unbalanced mind*. London: Wiedenfield & Nicolson.

Lehtinen, V., Aaltonen, J., Koffert, T., et al (2000) Two year outcome in first episode psychosis treated according to an integrated model. Is immediate neuroleptisation always needed? *European Psychiatry*, 15: 312-20.

Lehtonen, J. (1994) From dualism to psychobiological interaction, *British Journal of Psychiatry*, 164 (suppl 23), 20-6.

Lemert, E.M. (1967) *Human deviance, social problems and social control*. Englewood Cliffs: Prentice-Hall.

Lenzer, J. (2004) Bush plans to screen whole US population for mental illness. *British Medical Journal*, 328: 1458.

Leo, J.L. & Cohen, D.A. (2003) Broken brains or flawed studies? A critical review of ADHD neuroimaging research. *Journal of Mind and Behavior*, 24: 29-56.

Lewis, B.E. (2003) Prozac and the post-human politics of cyborgs. *Journal of Medical Humanities*, 24: 49-63.

Leys, R. (1999) *Guide to the Adolf Meyer collection*. Baltimore: John Hopkins www.medicalarchives.jhmi.edu/sgml/amg-d.htm.

Lidz, T. (1972) Schizophrenia, R.D. Laing and the contemporary treatment of psychosis. An interview with Robert Orrill & Robert Boyers. In: R. Boyers & R. Orrill (eds.) *Laing and anti-psychiatry*. Harmondsworth: Penguin.

Lidz, T., Cornelison, M.S.S., Fleck, S. & Terry, D. (1957) The intrafamilial environment of schizophrenic parents: II. Marital schism and marital skew. *American Journal of Psychiatry*, 114: 241-8.

Lieberman, J.A. (1999) Searching for the neuropathology of schizophrenia: Neuroimaging strategies and findings. *American Journal of Psychiatry*, 156: 1133-6.

Lief, A. (1948) (ed.) *The commonsense psychiatry of Dr Adolf Meyer*. New York: McGraw-Hill.

Link, B. & Cullen, F. (1990) The labeling theory of mental disorder: A review of the evidence. *Research in community and mental health*, 6: 75-105.

Lionells, M. (2000) The William Alanson White Institute yesterday, today and tomorrow. *American Psychoanalyst* www.wawhite.org/history/brief_history_WAWI.htm

Luhrmann, T.M. (2000) *Of two minds. The growing disorder in American psychiatry*. New York: Knopf.

Luk, S.L. & Leung, P.W.L. (1989) Connors teachers rating scale – a validity study in Hong Kong. *Journal of Child Psychology and Psychiatry*, **30**: 785-94.

Lynch, T. (2001) *Beyond Prozac. Healing mental suffering without drugs*. Dublin: Marino Books.

Macmurray, J. (1935) *Reason and emotion* London: Faber.

Maj, M. (2003). The effect of lithium in bipolar disorder: a review of recent research evidence. *Bipolar Disorders*, 5: 180-8.

Malt, U.F., Robak, O.H., Madsbu, H.-P., Bakke, O. & Loeb, M. (1999) The Norwegian naturalistic treatment study of depression in general practice (NORDEP) I: Randomised double blind study. *British Medical Journal,* 318: 1180-4.

Mamede, S. & Schmidt, H.G. (2004) The structure of reflective practice in medicine. *Medical Education,* 38: 1302-8.

Mann, E.M., Ikeda, Y., Mueller, C.W., et al (1992) Cross-cultural differences in rating hyperactive-disruptive behaviours in children. *American Journal of Psychiatry,* 149: 1539-42.

Marcuse, H. (1968) *One dimensional man.* London: Sphere.

Marinetto, M. (2003) Who wants to be an active citizen? The politics and practice of community involvement. *Sociology,* 37: 103–20.

Marshall, R. (1990) The genetics of schizophrenia: Axiom or hypothesis? In: R. Bentall (ed.) *Reconstructing schizophrenia.* London: Routledge.

Martin, J.P. (1984) *Hospitals in trouble.* Oxford: Blackwell.

Marx, O.M. (1972) Wilhelm Griesinger and the history of psychiatry: a reassessment. *Bulletin of the History of Medicine,* 46: 519-44.

Maudsley, G. & Strivens, J. (2000) Promoting professional knowledge, experiential learning and critical thinking for medical students. *Medical Education,* 34: 535-44.

Mazaide, M. (1989) Should adverse temperament matter to the clinician? An empirically based answer. In: G.A. Khonstaum, V.E. Bates & M.K. Rothbart (eds.) *Temperament in childhood.* New York: Wiley.

McCabe, R., Heath, C., Burns, T., et al (2002) Engagement of patients with psychosis in the consultation. *British Medical Journal,* 325: 1148-51.

McDowell, J. (1994) *Mind and world.* Harvard: University Press.

McGuiness, D. (1989) Attention deficit disorder, the emperor's new clothes, Animal 'Pharm' and other fiction. In: S. Fisher & R. Greenberg (eds.) *The limits of biological treatments for psychological distress: Comparisons with psychotherapy and placebo.* Hillsdale, N.J.: Lawrence Erlbaum Associates.

McKie, R. (2001) Revealed: The secret of human behaviour. *The Observer,* 11 February.

McWhinney, I.R. (1997) *A textbook of family medicine* (second edition). Oxford: Oxford University Press.

Medawar, C. (1997) The antidepressant web – Marketing depression and making medicines work. *International Journal of Risk & Safety in Medicine,* 10: 75-126.

Melander, H., Ahlqvist-Rastad, J., Meijer, G., Beerman, B. (2003) Evidence b(i)ased medicine-selective reporting from studies sponsored by pharmaceutical industry: review of studies in new drug applications. *British Medical Journal,* 326: 1171-3.

Menninger, K (1963) (with Mayman, M. & Pruyser, P.) *The vital balance.* New York: The Viking Press.

Meyer, A. (1896) Review of the fifth edition of Emil Kraepelin's textbook. *American Journal of Insanity,* 53: 298-302.

Meyer, A. (1906) Fundamental conceptions of dementia praecox. *British Medical Journal,* ii: 757-60.

Meyer, A. (1910) The dynamic interpretation of dementia praecox. *American Journal of Psychology,* 21: 385-403.

Meyer, A. (1912) Conditions for a home of psychology in the medical curriculum. *Journal of Abnormal Psychology,* 7: 313.

Meyer, A. (1957) *Psychobiology. A science of man* (comp. and ed. by E.E. Winters & A.M. Bowers). Springfield, Illinois: Charles C. Thomas.

MIMS Ireland (2000) September. Dublin: Medical Publications (Ireland).

Mind (1999) *Creating accepting communities: Report of the Mind inquiry into social exclusion and mental health problems.* London: Mind Publications.

Mind Freedom (2004) *Fast for freedom in mental health.* www.mindfreedom.org/mindfree dom/hungerstrike.shtml (accessed 1 March 2004).

Mitchell, R. (1993) *Crisis intervention in practice: The multidisciplinary team and the mental health social worker*. Aldershot: Avebury.

Moll, G., Hause, S., Ruther, E., Rothenberger, A. & Huether, G. (2001) Early methylphenidate administration to young rats causes a persistent reduction in the density of striatal dopamine transporters. *Journal of Child and Adolescent Psychopharmacology*, 11: 15-24.

Mollica, R.F. (1985) From Antonio Gramsci to Franco Basaglia: The theory and practice of the Italian psychiatric reform. *International Journal of Mental Health*, 14: 22-41.

Moncrieff, J. (1997). Lithium: Evidence reconsidered. *British Journal of Psychiatry*, 171: 113-19.

Moncrieff, J. (1999) An investigation into the precedents of modern drug treatment in psychiatry. *History of Psychiatry*, 10: 475-90.

Moncrieff, J. (2001). Are antidepressants overrated? A review of methodological problems in antidepressant trials. *Journal of Nervous and Mental Disease*, 189: 288-95.

Moncrieff, J. & Cohen, D. (2005) Re-thinking models of psychotropic drug action. *Psychotherapy and Psychosomatics*, 74: 145-53.

Moncrieff, J. & Crawford, M.J. (2001) British psychiatry in the 20th century – observations from a psychiatric journal. *Social Science & Medicine*, 53: 349-56.

Moncrieff, J. & Kirsch, I. (2005) Efficacy of antidepressants in adults. *British Medical Journal*, 331: 155-7.

Moncrieff, J., Wessely, S. & Hardy, R. (2004) Active placebos versus antidepressants for depression (Cochrane Review). In: *The Cochrane Library*, Issue 3, 2004. Chichester: Wiley.

Morgan, P. (1987) *Delinquent fantasies*. London: Temple Smith.

Morris, D. (2004) *The social inclusion programme*. London: NIMHE.

Morris, M. & MacPherson, R. (2001) Childhood 'risk characteristics' and the schizophrenia spectrum prodrome. *Irish Journal of Psychological Medicine*, 18: 72-4.

Morss, J.R. (1996) *Growing critical: Alternatives to developmental psychology*. London & New York: Routledge.

Mortimer, A.M. (1992) Phenomenology. Its place in schizophrenia research. *British Journal of Psychiatry*, 161: 293-7.

Mosher, L.R., Vallone, R. & Menn, A. (1995) The treatment of acute psychosis without neuroleptics: Six week psychopathology outcome data from the Soteria project. *International Journal of Social Psychiatry*, 41: 157-73.

Mother Jones (2002) Disorders made to order. *Mother Jones magazine*, July/August. www.motherjones.com

MTA Co-operative Group (1999) A 14 month randomized clinical trial of treatment strategies for attention deficit/hyperactivity disorder. *Archives of General Psychiatry*, 56: 1073-86.

Mullan, B. (1995) *Mad to be normal. Conversations with R.D. Laing*. London: Free Association.

Mullan, B. (1999) *R.D. Laing: A personal view*. London: Duckworth.

Mullender, A. & Ward, D. (1991) *Self-directed groupwork*. London : Whiting & Birch.

Muller-Hill, B. (1991) Psychiatry in the Nazi era. In: S. Block & P. Chodoff (eds.) *Psychiatric ethics*. New York: Oxford University Press.

Muncie, W. (1939) *Psychobiology and psychiatry. A textbook of normal and abnormal behaviour*. London: Henry Kimpton.

Murray, R. (1994) *The Independent*, 13 September.

Murray, R., Hill, P. & McGuffin, P. (1997) *The essentials of postgraduate psychiatry* (third edition). Cambridge: Cambridge University Press.

NAMI information leaflet (2003) *About mental illness*, www.nami.org (accessed 5 August 2005).

National Institute of Clinical Excellence (NICE) (2003) *Depression clinical guideline – first consultation.* www.nice.org.uk/Docref.asp?d=86349 (accessed on 19 September 2003).

National Institute for Clinical Excellence. (2004) *Management of depression in primary and secondary care* (clinical guideline 23). London: NICE

National Institute of Health Care Management (2002) *Prescription drug expenditures in 2001*, www.nichm.org.

National Institutes of Health (1998) *Consensus statement: Diagnosis and treatment of attention deficit hyperactivity disorders.* Rockville, M.D: National Institute of Mental Health.

Nirje, B. (1969) The normalisation principle and its human management implications. In: R.B. Kugel & W. Wolfensberger (eds.) *Changing patterns in services for the mentally retarded.* Washington D.C.: Presidential Committee on Mental Retardation.

Nuttall, J. (1970) *Bomb culture.* London: Paladin.

Oaks, D. (1998) A new proposal to Congress may mean daily psychiatric drug deliveries to your doorstep. *Dendron,* 41/42, 4-7. (The journal Dendron is published by the Support Coalition International.)

Obeyesekere, G. (1977) The theory and practice of psychological medicine in Ayurvedic tradition. *Culture Medicine and Psychiatry,* 1: 155-81.

Oh, V.M.S. (1994) The placebo effect: can we use it better? *British Medical Journal,* 309: 69-70.

Olfson, M., Marcus, S.C., Weissman, M.M. & Jensen, P.S. (2002) National trends in the use of psychotropic medications by children. *Journal of the American Academy of Child and Adolescent Psychiatry,* 41: 514-21.

O'Neill, J.R. (1980) Adolf Meyer and American psychiatry today. *American Journal of Psychiatry,* 137: 460-4.

Onyett, S. & Ford, R. (1996) Multidisciplinar community teams: Where is the wreckage? *Journal of Mental Health,* 5: 47-55.

Orion Pharma (1995) *Schizophrenia: A guide for families and carers.* Orion Pharma.

Pam. A. (1995) Introduction. In: C.A. Ross & A. Pam (eds.) *Pseudoscience in biological psychiatry: Blaming the body.* New York: Wiley.

Paykell, E.S. & Priest, R.G. (1992) Recognition and management of depression in general practice: consensus statement. *British Medical Journal,* 305: 1198-202.

Paykel, E.S., Hart, D. & Priest, R.G. (1998) Changes in public attitudes to depression during the Defeat Depression Campaign. *British Journal of Psychiatry,* 173: 519-22

Peay, J. (1996) (ed.) *Inquiries after homicide.* London: Duckworth.

Perkins, R., Buckfield, R. & Choy, D. (1997) Access to employment: A supported employment project to enable mental health service users to obtain jobs within mental health teams. *Journal of Mental Health,* 6: 307-18.

Pharmaceutical Marketing (2001) Practical Guides: Medical Education parts I & II. *Pharmaceutical Marketing.* (Available on request from www.pmlive.com)

Pickles, A., Rowe, R., Simonoff, E., et al (2001) Child psychiatric symptoms and psychosocial impairment: relationship and prognostic significance. *British Journal of Psychiatry,* 179: 230-53.

Pincus, H.A., Tanielian, T.L. & Marcus, S.C. (1998) Prescribing trends in psychotropic medications. *Journal of the Aerican Medical Association,* 279: 526-31.

Porter, R. (1987) *A social history of madness. Stories of the insane.* London : Weidenfeld & Nicolson.

Posternak, M., Zimmerman, M., Keitner, G.I. & Miller, I.W. (2002) A re-evaluation of exclusion criteria uses in antidepressant efficacy trials. *American Journal of Psychiatry,* 159: 191-200.

Prien, R.F., Caffey, E.M., Jr. & Klett, C.J. (1972). Comparison of lithium carbonate and chlorpromazine in the treatment of mania. Report of the Veterans Administration and

National Institute of Mental Health Collaborative Study Group. *Archives General Psychiatry*, **26**: 146-53.

Priest, R.G., Vize, C., Roberts, A. et al (1996) Lay people's attitudes to treatment of depression: results of opinion poll for Defeat Depression Campaign just before its launch. *British Medical Journal*, 313: 858-9.

Prout, A. & James, A. (1997) A new paradigm for the sociology of childhood? Provenance, promise and problems. In: A. James & A. Prout (eds.) *Constructing and re-constructing childhood: Contemporary issues in the sociological study of childhood*. London: Falmer Press.

Public Citizen (2002) America's other drug problem: a briefing book on the prescription drug debate. www.citizen.org/rxfacts.

Rahman, A. (1993) *People's self-development*. London: Zed Press.

Ramon, S. (1985) *Psychiatry in Britain: Meaning and policy*. London: Croom Helm.

Ramon, S. (1989) The impact of the Italian psychiatric reforms on North American and British professionals. *The International Journal of Social Psychiatry*, 35: 120-7.

Ramon, S. (1991) (ed.) *Beyond community care: Normalisation and integration work*. London: Macmillan.

Ramon, S. (1992) (ed.) *Psychiatric hospitals closure: Myths and reality*. London: Chapman Hall.

Ramon, S. (2000) (ed.) *A stakeholder's approach to innovation in mental health services: A reader for the 21st century*. Brighton: Pavilion Publishing.

Ramon, S. (2003) (ed.) *Users researching health and social care: An empowering agenda?* Birmingham: Venture Press.

Ramon, S. (2005) Approaches to risk in mental health: A multidisciplinary discourse. In: J. Tew (ed.) *Social perspectives in mental health: Developing social models to understanding and work with mental distress*. London: Jessica Kingsley, pp. 184-99.

Ramon, S. & Williams, J. (2005) (eds.) *Mental health at the crossroads: The promise of the psychosocial approach*. Aldershot: Ashgate.

Rapaport. J. (2005) The informal caring experience: Issues and dilemmas. In: S. Ramon & J. Williams (2005) (eds.) *Mental health at the crossroads: The promise of the psychosocial approach*. Aldershot: Ashgate, pp. 155-70.

Rapoport, J.L., Buchsbaum, M.S., Zahn, T., et al (1978) Dextroamphetamine: Cognitive and behavioural effects in normal prepubertal boys. *Science, 199*: 560-3.

Rapoport, J.L., Buchsbaum, M.S., Zahn, T., et al (1980) Dextroamphetamine: Its cognitive and behavioural effect in normal and hyperactive boys and normal men. *Archives of General Psychiatry, 37*: 933-43.

Rapp, C.A. (1992) The strengths perspective of case management with persons suffering from severe mental illness. In: D. Saleeby (ed.) *The strengths approach in social work*. New York: Longman, pp. 45-58.

Ravenel, D.B. (2002) A new behavioral approach for ADD/ADHD and behavioral management without medication. *Ethical Human Sciences and Services, 4*: 93-106.

Redler, L. (1976) Anti-psychiatry (letter). *The New Review, 3*: 71-2.

Rie, H., Rie, E., Stewart, S. & Anbuel, J. (1976) Effects of Ritalin on underachieving children: A replication. *American Journal of Orthopsychiatry, 45*: 313-32.

Rioch, M. (1986) Fifty years at the Washington school of psychiatry. *Psychiatry, 49*: 33-44.

Robin, A.L. & Barkley, R.A. (1998) *ADHD in adolescents: Diagnosis and treatment*. New York: Guildford.

Rogers, A. & Pilgrim, D. (2001) *A sociology of mental illness*. Milton Keynes: The Open University Press.

Rogers, A., Day, J. C., Williams, B., et al (1998) The meaning and management of neuroleptic medication: a study of patients with a diagnosis of schizophrenia. *Social Science Medicine, 47*: 1313-23.

Rose, D. (2000) A year of care. *OpenMind, 106*: 8-9.

Rose, N. (1979) The psychological complex: mental measurement and social administration. *Ideology and Consciousness*, 4: 5–68.

Rose, N. (1996) The death of the social? Re-figuring the territory of government. *Economy and Society*, 25: 327–56.

Rose, S. (1997) When making things simple does not give the right explanation. *Times Higher Education Supplement*, 5 September, pp. 16-17.

Rose, S. (1998) *Lifelines: Biology, freedom, determinism*. London: Penguin.

Rose, S. (2005) *The 21ˢᵗ century brain: Explaining, mending and manipulating the mind*. London: Jonathan Cape.

Rose, S., Lewontin, R.C., & Kamin, L.J. (1990) *Not in our genes*. Harmondsworth: Penguin.

Rosenhan, D.L. (1973) On being sane in insane places. *Science*, 179: 250-8.

Roth, M. (1973) Psychiatry and its critics. *British Journal of Psychiatry*, 122: 373-8.

Roth, M. & Kroll, J. (1986) *The reality of mental illness*. Cambridge: Cambridge University Press.

Royal College of Psychiatrists (2002) *Antidepressant factsheet*. London: Royal College of Psychiatrists.

Royal Commission (1926) *Report of the Royal Commission on lunacy and mental disorders* (Cmd. 2700). London: Stationery Office.

Rush, B. (1962) *Medical inquiries and observations upon the diseases of the mind* (Original edition 1812). New York: Hafner.

Sabshin, M. (1990) Turning points in twentieth-century American psychiatry. *American Journal of Psychiatry*, 147: 1267-74.

Sachs, W. (1992) *The developmental dictionary*. London: Zed Press.

Safer, D.J. (2002) Design and reporting modifications in industry sponsored comparative psychopharmacology trials. *Journal of Nervous and Mental Disease*, 190: 583-92.

Saleeby, D. (1992) (ed.) *The strength approach in social work*. New York: Longman.

Sannerud, C. & Feussner, G. (2000) Is Ritalin an abused drug? Does it meet the criteria of a schedule II substance? In: L.L. Greenhill & B.B. Osman (eds.) *Ritalin: Theory and practice*. New York: Mary Ann Liebert.

Sarbin, T. (1991) The social construction of schizophrenia. In: W. Flack, D. Miller & M. Wiener (eds.) *What is schizophrenia?* New York: Springer-Verlag.

Sartorius, N., Gulbinat, W., Harrison, G., et al (1996) Long-term follow-up of schizophrenia in 16 countries. A description of the International Study of Schizophrenia conducted by the World Health Organization. *Social Psychiatry and Psychiatric Epidemiology* 31: 249-58.

Sartre, J-P. (1957) *The transcendence of the ego* (trans. F. Williams & R. Kirkpatrick). New York: Noonday Press.

Sartre, J-P. (1989) *Vérité et existence*. Paris: Gallimard.

Sayce, L. (2000) *From psychiatric patient to citizen: Overcoming discrimination and social exclusion*. Macmillan Press: London.

Schachar, R. & Tannock, R. (2002) Syndromes of hyperactivity and attention deficit. In: M. Rutter & E. Taylor (eds.) *Child and adolescent psychiatry* (fourth edition). Oxford: Blackwell.

Schachter, H., Pham, B., King, J., et al (2001). How efficacious and safe is short-acting methylphenidate for the treatment of attention-deficit disorder in children and adolescents? A meta-analysis. *Canadian Medical Association Journal*, 165: 1475-88.

Schatzman, M. (1972) Madness and morals. In: R. Boyers & R. Orrill (eds.) *Laing and anti-psychiatry*. Harmondsworth: Penguin.

Scheff, T.J. (1999) *Being mentally ill: A sociological theory* (third edition). New York: Aldine de Gruyter.

Scheper-Hughes, N. & Lovell, A.M. (1987) (eds.) *Psychiatry inside out: Selected writings of Franco Basaglia*. New York: Columbia University Press.

Scheper-Hughes, N. & Stein, H.F. (1987) Child abuse and the unconscious in American popular culture. In: N. Scheper-Hughes (ed.) *Child survival*. New York: D. Reidel Publishing.

Schneider, K. (1959) *Clinical psychopathology* (trans M.W. Hamilton). London: Grune & Stratton.

Schon, D. (1987) *Educating the reflective practitioner*. San Franscisco: Jossey-Bass.

Schooler, N.R., Goldberg, S.C., Boothe, H. & Cole J.O. (1967) One year after discharge: community adjustment of schizophrenic patients. *American Journal of Psychiatry*, 123: 986-95.

Schore, A. (2001) The effects of early relational trauma on right brain development, affect regulation, and infant mental health. *Infant Mental Health Journal*, 22: 201-69.

Scull, A. (1979) *Decarceration*. Cambridge: Cambridge Polity Press.

Scull, A. (1993) *The most solitary of afflictions: Madness and society in Britain 1700-1900*. New Haven: Yale University Press.

Scull, A. (1994) Somatic treatments and the historiography of psychiatry. *History of Psychiatry*, 5: 1-12.

Scull, A. (2005) *Madhouse: A tragic tale of megalomania and modern medicine*. London: Yale University Press.

Seabrook, J. (1982) *Working class childhood: An oral history*. London: Gollancz.

Searles, H.F. (1959) The effort to drive the other person crazy; an element in the aetiology and psychotherapy of schizophrenia. *British Journal of Medical Psychology*, 32: 1-18.

Secker, J., Membrey, H., Grove, B., & Seebohm, P. (2002) Recoverying from illness or recovering your life? Implications of clinical vs. social models of recovery from mental illness for employment support services. *Disability & Society*, 17: 403-28.

Sedgwick, P. (1972) R.D. Laing: self, symptom and society. In: R. Boyers & R. Orrill. (eds.) *Laing and anti-psychiatry*. Harmondsorth: Penguin.

Sedgwick, P. (1981) The grapes of Roth. Book review of *Critical Psychiatry: The Politics of Mental Health* by David Ingleby (ed.). *New Society*, 30 April 1981 (also available at www.criticalpsychiatry.co.uk/Grapes.htm).

Sedley, B. (2000) Why change anything? In: S. Ramon (ed.) *A stakeholder's approach to innovation in metal health services: A reader for the 21st century*. Brighton: Pavilion, pp. 47-59.

Shen, Y.C., Wong, Y.F. & Yang, X.L. (1985) An epidemiological investigation of minimal brain dysfunction in six elementary schools in Beijing. *Journal of Child Psychology and Psychiatry*, 26: 777-88.

Shepherd, M. (1976) Definition, classification and nomenclature: A clinical overview. In: D.Kemali, G. Bartholini & D. Richer (eds.). *Schizophrenia today*. Oxford: Pergamon.

Shepherd, M. (1986) A representative psychiatrist: the career, contributions and legacies of Sir Aubrey Lewis. *Psychological Medicine Monograph Supplement 10*.

Sherman, N. (1989) *The fabric of character: Aristotle's theory of virtue*. Oxford: Clarendon.

Shorter, E. (1997) *A History of psychiatry*. New York: Wiley.

Silberg, J., Rutter, M., Meyer, J., et al (1996) Genetic and environmental influences on the covariation between hyperactivity and conduct disturbance in juvenile twins. *Journal of Child Psychology and Psychiatry*, 37: 803-16.

Singer, M.T. & Wynne, L.C. (1965) Thought disorder and family relations of schizophrenics. IV. Results and implications. *Archives of General Psychiatry 12*: 201-12.

Skelton, C. (2001) *Schooling the boys: Masculinities and primary education*. Buckingham: Open University Press.

Skrabanek, P. (1984) Biochemistry of schizophrenia: a pseudoscientific model. *Integrative Psychiatry*, 2: 224-8.

Slater, E. & Roth, M. (1969) *Clinical psychiatry* (third edition). London: Bailliere, Tindall & Cassell.

Sluga, H (2002) Frege on the indefinability of truth. In: H. Reck (ed.) *From Frege to Wittgenstein*. Oxford: University Press.

Smail, D. (1996) J. Richard Marshall. *Clinical Psychology Forum*, 95: 14-16.

Smith, N.H. (2002) *Reading McDowell on mind and world*. London: Routledge.

Social Exclusion Unit (2004) *Mental health and social exclusion*. London: Office of the Deputy Prime Minister (available online at: www.publications.odpm.goc.uk/).

Sonuga-Barke, E.J.S., Minocha, K., Taylor, E.A. & Sandberg, S. (1993) Inter-ethnic bias in teachers' ratings of childhood hyperactivity. *British Journal of Developmental Psychology*, 11: 187-200.

Spencer, T., Biederman, J., Wilens, T., et al (1996) Pharmacotherapy of attention deficit hyperactivity disorder across the life cycle. *Journal of the American Academy of Child and Adolescent Psychiatry*, 35: 409-32.

Spitzer, R.L. (1976) More on pseudoscience in science and the case for psychiatric diagnosis. *Archives of General Psychiatry*, 33: 459-70.

Spitzer, R.L. & Fleiss, J.L. (1974) A reanalysis of the reliability of psychiatric diagnosis. *British Journal of Psychiatry*, 125: 341-7.

Spizer, R.L., Endicott, J. & Robins, E. (1975) *Research diagnostic criteria (RDC) for a selected group of functional disorders*. New York: New York State Psychiatric Institute.

Sproson, E.J., Chantrey, J., Hollis, C., Marsden, C.A. & Fonel, K.C. (2001) Effect of repeated methylphenidate administration on presynaptic dopamine and behavior in young adult rats. *Journal of Psychopharmacology*, 15: 67-75.

Stanley, N., Manthorpe, J. & Penhale, B. (1999) (eds.) *Institutional abuse*. London: Routledge.

Stewart, M., Brown, J.B., Weston, W.W., et al (2003) *Patient-centred medicine. Transforming the clinical method* (second edition). Abingdon: Radcliffe Medical Press.

Stuttaford, T. (1999) (writing about depression) *The Times*, 25 May.

Suvannathat, C., Bhanthumnavin, D., Bhuapirom, L. & Keats, D.M. (1985) *Handbook of Asian child development and child rearing practices*. Bangkok: Srina Kharinwirot University.

Swain, J., Finkelstein, V., French, S. & Oliver, M. (1996) *Disabling barriers – Enabling environments*. Milton Keynes: The Open University.

Swazey, J. (1974) *Chlorpromazine in psychiatry*. Cambridge, MA: Massachusetts Institute of Technology.

Szasz, T.S. (1972) *The myth of mental illness*. London: Paladin.

Szasz, T.S. (1976) Anti-psychiatry: The paradigm of the plundered mind. *The New Review*, 3: 3-14.

Szasz, T.S. (1987) *Insanity: The idea and its consequences*. New York: Wiley.

Szasz, T.S. (1999) *Ideology and insanity*. Syracuse: Syracuse University Press.

Szasz, T.S. (2001) *Pharmacracy. Medicine and Politics in America*. London: Praeger.

Szasz, T.S. (2004a) 'Knowing what ain't so': RD Laing and Thomas Szasz. *Psychoanalytic Review*, 91: 331-46.

Szasz, T.S (2004b) Psychiatric fraud and force: A critique of E. Fuller Torrey. *Journal of Humanistic Psychology*, 44: 416-30.

Tantam, D. (1991) The anti-psychiatry movement. In: G.E. Berrios & H. Freeman (eds.) *150 Years of British Psychiatry, 1841-1991*. London: Gaskell.

Taylor, E. & Hemsley, R. (1995) Treating hyperkinetic disorders in childhood. *British Medical Journal*, 310: 1617-18.

Taylor, E. (1994) Syndromes of attention deficit and overactivity. In: M. Rutter, E. Taylor & L. Hersov (eds.) *Child and adolescent psychiatry, Modern approaches* (Third edition). Oxford: Blackwell Scientific Publications.

Taylor, E., Schachar, R., Thorley, G., et al (1987) Which boys respond to stimulant medication? A controlled trial of Methylphenidate in boys with disruptive behaviour. *Psychological Medicine*, 17: 121-43.

Tew, J. (2005) (ed.) *Social perspectives in mental health: Developing social models to understand and work with mental distress.* London: Jessica Kingsley.

The Independent (1998) 19 February.

Thomas S. Szasz Cybercenter for Liberty and Responsibility (2004) www.szasz.com (accessed 6 June 2004).

Thomas, A. & Chess, S. (1977) *Temperament and development.* New York: Brunner-Mazel.

Thomas, P. (1997) *The dialectics of schizophrenia.* London: Free Association Books.

Thomas, P. & Bracken, P. (2004) Critical psychiatry in practice. *Advances in Psychiatric Treatment,* 10: 361–70.

Thomas, P., Bracken, P. & Leudar, I. (2004) Hearing Voices: A phenomenological-hermeneutic approach. *Cognitive Neuropsychiatry,* 9: 13–23.

Thomas, P., Bracken, P., Cutler, P., et al (2005) Challenging the globalisation of biomedical psychiatry. *Journal of Public Mental Health,* 4: 23-32

Thomas, P. & Moncrieff, J. (1999) Joined-up thinking. *Health Matters* **39**: www. healthmatters.org.uk/stories/pthomas.html (accessed 9 September 2004).

Timimi S. (2002a) *Pathological child psychiatry and the medicalisation of childhood.* London: Brunner-Routledge.

Timimi, S. (2002b) The politics of prescribing psychotropic medication to children and adolescents. *Postgraduate Doctor,* 18: 175-7.

Timimi, S. (2004) Rethinking childhood depression. *British Medical Journal,* 329: 1394-6.

Timimi, S. (2005) *Naughty boys: Anti-social behaviour, ADHD and the role of culture.* Basingstoke: Palgrave MacMillan.

Timimi, S. & Taylor, E. (2004) ADHD is best understood as a cultural construct. *British Journal of Psychiatry,* 184: 8-9.

Timms, N. (1964) *The history of psychiatric social work.* London: Routledge & Kegan Paul.

Toren, N. (1972) *Social work: The case of a semi-profession.* London: Sage.

Torrey, E.F. (1974) *The death of psychiatry.* New York: Penguin.

Torrey, E.F. (1983) *Surviving schizophrenia: A manual for families, consumers, and providers.* New York: Harper & Row.

Torrey, E.F. & Kress, K.J. (2004) *The new neurobiology of severe psychiatric disorders and its implications for laws governing involuntary commitment and treatment.* University of Iowa Legal Studies Research Paper No. 04-04. http://ssrn.com/abstract=634243

Torrey, E.F. & Miller, J. (2001) *The invisible plague: The rise of mental illness from 1750 to the present.* New Brunswick: Rutgers University Press

Trevillion, S. (1992) *Caring in the community: A networking approach to community partnership.* Harlow: Longman.

Turkle, S. (2004) French anti-psychiatry. In: D. Ingleby (ed.) *Critical psychiatry: The politics of mental health.* London: Free Association Books.

Turner, T. (1998) Summer edition of *Community Mental Health.*

Tyrer, P. (1996) Co-morbidity or consanguinity. *British Journal of Psychiatry,* **168**: 669-71.

Tyrer, P., Duggan, C. & Coid, J. (2003) Ramifications of personality disorder in clinical practice *British Journal of Psychiatry* 182: (suppl. 44): s1-s2.

US Department of Health and Human Services (1999) *Mental Health: A Report of the Surgeon General—Executive Summary.* Rockville, MD: US Department of Health and Human Services, Substance Abuse and Mental Health Services Administration, Center for Mental Health Services, National Institutes of Health, National Institute of Mental Health.

Unsworth, C. (1987) *The politics of mental health legislation.* Oxford: Clarendon Press.

van Dijk, R. (1998) Culture as excuse. The failures of health care to migrants in the Netherlands. In: S. Van der Geest & A. Rienks (eds.) *The art of medical anthropology: Readings.* Amsterdam: Spinhuis, pp. 243-51.

Viguera, A.C., Baldessarini, R.J., Hegarty, J.D., et al (1997). Clinical risk following abrupt and gradual withdrawal of maintenance neuroleptic treatment. *Archives of General Psychiatry*, 54: 49-55.

Viguera, A.C., Baldessarini, R.J., & Friedberg, J. (1998). Discontinuing antidepressant treatment in major depression. *Harvard Review Psychiatry*, 5: 293-306.

Volkow, N.D., Ding, Y.S., Fowler, J.S., et al (1995) Is methylphenidate like cocaine? *Archives of General Psychiatry*, 52: 456-63.

Wagner, L.C. & King, M. (2005) Existential needs of people with psychotic disorders in Porto Alegre, Brazil. *British Journal of Psychiatry*, 186: 141-5.

Walker, S. (2003) Social work and child mental health: Psycho-social principles in community practice. *British Journal of Social Work*, 33: 673-87.

Wallace, M. (1985) The tragedy of schizophrenia. *The Times*, December.

Wallcraft, J. (2003) (with Read, J. & Sweeney, A.) *On our own terms: Users and survivors of mental health services working together for support and change.* London: Sainsbury Centre.

Wallcraft, J. (2005) Recovery from Mental Breakdown. In: J. Tew (ed.) *Social perspectives in mental health: Developing social models to understand and work with mental distress.* London: Jessica Kingsley, pp. 200-15.

Weinman-Lear, M. (1963) *The child worshipers.* New York: Pocket.

Weis, G., Kruger, E., Danielson, U. & Elman, M. (1975) Effect of long term treatment of hyperactive children with methylphenidate. *Canadian Medical Association Journal*, 112: 159-65.

Wessely, S. (1996) The rise of counselling and the return of alienism. *British Medical Journal*, 313: 158-60.

White, W.A. (1933) *Forty years of pychiatry.* New York: Nervous & Mental Disease Publication Co.

Whittington, C.J., Kendall, T., Fonagy, P., et al (2004). Selective serotonin reuptake inhibitors in childhood depression: systematic review of published versus unpublished data. *Lancet*, 363: 1341-5.

Wickes-Nelson, R. & Israel, A. (2002) *Behaviour disorders of childhood.* London: Pearson Higher Education.

Wilkinson, R.G. (1996) *Unhealthy societies: The afflications of inequality.* London: Routledge.

Williams, B. (2002) *Truth and truthfulness.* Princeton: University Press.

Williams, B., Thomas, P., Cattell, D., et al (1999) Exploring 'person-centredness': User perspectives on a model of social psychiatry. *Health and Social Care in the Community*, 7: 475-82.

Williams, J. (2005) Living with trauma. In: S. Ramon & J. Williams (eds.) *Mental health at the crossroads: The promise of the psychosocial approach.* Aldershot: Ashgate, pp.171-85

Williams, L (1992) Torture and the torturer. *The Psychologist*, 5: 305-8.

Williams, M. (1999) *Wittgenstein, mind and meaning.* London: Routledge.

Wilson, M. (1993) DSM-III and the transformation of American psychiatry: a history. *American Journal of Psychiatry*, 150: 399-410.

Winn, M. (1984) *Children without childhood.* Harmondsworth: Penguin.

Winokur, G. (1975). The Iowa 500: heterogeneity and course in manic-depressive illness (bipolar). *Comprehensive Psychiatry*, 16: 125-31.

Winters, E.E. (1950, 1951) *The collected papers of Adolf Meyer* (four volumes). Baltimore: Johns Hopkins Press.

Wittgenstein, L. (1980) *Remarks on the philosophy of psychology* (vol. 2). Oxford: Blackwell.

Wolfensberger, W. (1972) *The principle of normalisation in human services.* Toronto: National Institute on Mental Retardation.

Wolfensberger, W. (1983) Social role valorisation: A proposed new term for the principle of normalisation. *Mental Retardation* 21: 234-39.

Wolfensberger, W. (1989) Self-injurious behavior, behavioristic responses and social role valorisation: A reply to Mulick and Kedesdy. *Mental Retardation*, 27: 181-4.

Wolfenstein, M. (1955) Fun morality: An analysis of recent child-training literature. In: M. Mead & M. Wolfenstein (eds.) *Childhood in contemporary cultures.* Chicago: The University of Chicago Press.

Wong, I.C., Murray, M.L., Camilleri-Novak, D. & Stephens, P. (2004) Increased prescribing trends of paediatric psychotropic medications. *Archives of Disease in Childhood*, 89: 1131-2.

World Health Organisation (1953) *Expert committee on mental health: Third report.* Geneva: WHO.

Wortis, J. (1986) Adolph Meyer: Some recollections and impressions. *British Journal of Psychiatry*, 149: 677- 81.

Wright, O. (2003) Ritalin use and abuse fears. *The Times*, 28 July.

Yale Bulletin and Calendar (2001) Dr. Theodore Lidz, a noted specialist on schizophrenia, dies. *Yale Bulletin and Calendar*, 2 March. www.yale.edu/opa/v29.n21/story14.html (accessed 27 July 2004).

Yelloly, M. & Henkel, M. (1995) (eds.) *Learning and teaching in social work: Towards reflective practice.* London: Jessica Kingsley.

Zelizer, V.A. (1985) *Pricing the priceless child: The changing social value of children.* New York: Basic Books Inc.

Zito, J.M., Safer, D.J., Dosreis, S., et al (2000) Trends in prescribing of psychotropic medication in pre-schoolers. *Journal of the American Medical Association*, 283: 1025-30.

Zohar, D. (1991) *The quantum self.* London: Flamingo.

Zubin, J. & Spring, B. (1977) Vulnerability – a new view of schizophrenia. *Journal of Abnormal Psychology*, 86: 103-26.

Zuckerman, M. (1975) Dr. Spock: The confidence man. In: S. Kaplan & C. Rosenberg (eds.) *The family in history.* Philadelphia: University of Pennsylvania Press.

Zwi, M., Ramchandani, P. & Joughlin, C. (2000) Evidence and belief in ADHD. *British Medical Journal*, 321: 975-6.

Index

ADHD (attention-deficit/hyperactivity disorder), 13, 196, 197, 198, 199, 200, 227, 229, 232, 237, 241, 245, 247

American Psychiatric Association, 12, 36, 68, 185, 215, 227, 231
   DSM (Diagnostic and Statistical Manual), 36, 68, 69, 75, 84, 85, 86, 153, 154, 162, 178, 185, 218, 233, 236, 246

anti-psychiatry, 4, 5, 6, 7, 8, 9, 11, 13, 19, 20, 21, 24, 25, 26, 27, 28, 29, 30, 31, 32, 35, 36, 37, 38, 39, 41, 42, 43, 63, 64, 126, 129, 134, 155, 156, 162, 163, 165, 166, 171, 187, 209, 210, 212, 218, 229, 230, 235, 237, 242, 243, 244, 245

Arbours Association, 27, 28, 39, 129

Basaglia, F., 32, 33, 34, 39, 228, 239, 242
   Psichiatria Democratica, 32, 33

Bateson, G., 20, 21, 228

Beers, C., 170, 173, 228

Berke, J., 20, 27, 37, 39, 227, 228, 232

biochemical imbalance, 9, 87, 89, 97, 101, 110

biomedical model, 11, 13, 36, 38, 69, 81, 82, 85, 95, 96, 98, 140, 145, 165, 185, 186, 187, 196, 209, 212, 215, 217, 218, 221, 223, 224, 225

biopsychological approach, 38, 165

child psychiatry, xii, 13, 190, 196, 205, 245

childhood depression, 200, 201

Cooper, D., 7, 19, 20, 21, 24, 25, 26, 28, 29, 36, 37, 39, 41, 42, 46, 63, 64, 200, 212, 230, 231, 232, 237
   Psychiatry and anti-psychiatry, 19

Critical Mental Health Forum, 213

critical psychiatry, 3, 4, 5, 6, 7, 8, 9, 11, 12, 13, 14, 15, 42, 45, 46, 49, 61, 62, 65, 70, 71, 78, 155, 156, 163, 187, 210, 211, 212, 213, 214, 215, 216, 217, 218, 219, 220, 223, 224, 231, 235

Critical Psychiatry Network, 6, 213, 214, 215, 232

critical theory, 4, 210, 212, 213

Dialectics of Liberation conference, 20, 42

drugs, 9, 10, 44, 89, 98, 99, 104, 107, 108, 113, 115, 116, 117, 118, 119, 120, 121, 123, 124, 125, 126, 128, 129, 130, 131, 132, 153, 154, 193, 195, 200, 230, 233, 236, 237
   antidepressant medication, 99, 100, 104, 105, 106, 107, 120, 122, 225, 234, 236, 238, 239, 240, 246

antipsychotic medication, 10,
116, 117, 118, 119, 123,
130
lithium, 10, 111, 119, 120,
224, 228, 235, 237, 240
neuroleptic medication, 131,
241, 246
Ritalin, 12, 13, 116, 120,
199, 200, 229, 233, 234,
241, 242, 247
ECT, 41, 81, 87, 98, 115, 125,
154, 219
Feuchtersleben, E. von, 168,
186, 229
Foucault, M., 7, 8, 26, 32, 43,
47, 48, 49, 51, 55, 70, 151,
160, 212, 232, 234
Foudraine, J., 6, 7, 32, 232, 235
Freud, S., 10, 48, 49, 50, 51, 52,
57, 153, 157, 170, 179, 185,
229, 233
genetic causation of mental
illness, 91, 92, 93, 235, 243
globalisation, 8, 61, 72, 162,
245
Ingleby, D., 3, 4, 5, 8, 12, 31,
36, 61, 66, 67, 70, 75, 82, 95,
98, 157, 215, 230, 234, 235,
236, 243, 245
Jones, M., 19, 27, 33, 39, 62
Dingleton hospital, 27, 33,
39
Kingsley Hall, 20, 22, 27, 28,
29, 129, 236
Kraepelin, E., 36, 72, 169, 170,
176, 177, 178, 180, 236, 238
Laing, R.D.,
Knots, 23, 236
*Sanity, madness and the
family*, 35
The divided self, 21, 22, 236

The politics of experience,
22, 212, 236
Wisdom, madness and folly,
24, 236
medication, 9, 10, 12, 14, 39,
69, 81, 87, 88, 89, 90, 95, 99,
100, 102, 103, 104, 105, 107,
109, 110, 112, 115, 156, 189,
195, 196, 197, 198, 199, 203,
205, 206, 214, 220, 223, 224,
225, 234, 236, 241, 244, 245,
247
Mental Health Act, 10, 11, 37,
127, 128, 140, 141, 144, 145,
158, 213, 218, 227, 231
mental hygiene, 64, 170, 173,
182
Meyer, A., 12, 38, 165, 166,
170, 171, 172, 173, 174, 175,
176, 177, 178, 179, 180, 181,
182, 183, 184, 185, 186, 187,
209, 218, 233, 237, 238, 240,
243, 246, 247
pharmaceutical industry, 10, 65,
97, 102, 108, 121, 123, 124,
132, 149, 150, 162, 183, 195,
204, 205, 214, 228, 238
Philadelphia Association, 7, 20,
22, 27, 28, 29, 39
placebo, 9, 14, 103, 104, 105,
118, 119, 120, 124, 130, 199,
214, 220, 228, 232, 238, 240
postmodern, 11, 154, 162, 193,
229
postpsychiatry, 11, 150, 156,
157, 158, 163
power, 3, 7, 8, 24, 30, 37, 42,
43, 47, 48, 49, 50, 53, 55, 57,
58, 62, 63, 67, 68, 69, 70, 71,
77, 78, 101, 102, 112, 123,
132, 139, 140, 144, 145, 153,
154, 160, 161, 164, 189, 192,

194, 204, 210, 212, 218, 220, 227, 229, 232
pragmatism, 39, 135, 170, 180
psychiatric diagnosis, 9, 30, 35, 36, 66, 82, 85, 86, 87, 100, 134, 174, 176, 177, 185, 186, 218, 244
psychoanalysis, 7, 8, 10, 45, 46, 47, 51, 52, 53, 54, 57, 62, 67, 125, 126, 135, 152, 156, 170, 174, 178, 179, 180, 181, 182, 185, 218, 223, 230, 233, 234
psychobiology, 170, 171, 175, 180, 181, 184, 185, 187, 209, 218, 238, 239
Redler, L., 20, 27, 28, 29, 37, 39, 233, 241
Rosenhan, D., 35, 36, 242
Roth, M., 3, 5, 30, 31, 32, 69, 180, 242, 243
Royal College of Psychiatrists, 4, 14, 30, 69, 116, 213, 233, 235, 242

Scheff, T., 31, 34, 35, 242
Sedgwick, P., 3, 5, 23, 69, 243
Social Perspectives Network, 11, 231
social work, 11, 133, 134, 136, 137, 139, 140, 141, 142, 143, 145, 146, 147, 182, 212, 227, 229, 241, 242, 245, 247
Szasz, T., 4, 5, 20, 28, 29, 30, 31, 37, 38, 39, 41, 42, 66, 168, 221, 236, 237, 244, 245
  insanity defence, 29, 30
  myth of mental illness, 28, 29, 244
Tavistock clinic, 5, 134
transcultural psychiatry, 8, 61, 71, 74, 76, 78
users of mental health services, 11, 78, 97, 109, 129, 138, 139, 142, 143, 147, 148, 155, 158, 162, 182, 228